T0202057

Spanked

How Hitting Our Children Is Harming Ourselves

Christina L. Erickson, PhD

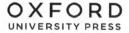
OXFORD
UNIVERSITY PRESS

OXFORD
UNIVERSITY PRESS

Oxford University Press is a department of the University of Oxford. It furthers
the University's objective of excellence in research, scholarship, and education
by publishing worldwide. Oxford is a registered trade mark of Oxford University
Press in the UK and certain other countries.

Published in the United States of America by Oxford University Press
198 Madison Avenue, New York, NY 10016, United States of America.

Library of Congress Cataloging-in-Publication Data
Names: Erickson, Christina L., author.
Title: Spanked : how hitting our children is harming ourselves / Christina L. Erickson, PhD.
Description: New York, NY : Oxford University Press, [2022] |
Includes bibliographical references and index.
Identifiers: LCCN 2022018788 (print) | LCCN 2022018789 (ebook) |
ISBN 9780197518236 (hardback) | ISBN 9780197518250 (epub)
Subjects: LCSH: Corporal punishment of children. | Discipline of children. |
Child psychology. | Children and violence.
Classification: LCC HQ770.4 .E738 2022 (print) | LCC HQ770.4 (ebook) |
DDC 649/.64—dc23/eng/20220518
LC record available at https://lccn.loc.gov/2022018788
LC ebook record available at https://lccn.loc.gov/2022018789

DOI: 10.1093/oso/9780197518236.001.0001

1 3 5 7 9 8 6 4 2

Printed by Sheridan Books, Inc., United States of America

For Honchie. Always.

Unless we cop out in some way, the challenge to bring more of ourselves into life is the healthiest kind of problem we can have. It looks different for different ages—a boy learns to be a friend, and then to be a husband and a father, and it is not ended then. Each stage has a cluster of challenges that demand something more of him that is clean and true. We go through life moderating our own resources, building new dimensions of ourselves on the structures we have just laid down. The everyday problems come in connection with growing. These are always an invitation to develop and come to grips with the difficulties that each new moment presents. We don't really get through life by solving problems in a final way but by responding more adequately as we move along.

Eugene Kennedy, *Living with Everyday Problems*[1]

Contents

Preface

The first time I remember wanting to use physical punishment—what most would call a spanking—with my two daughters was when they were around 2 and 4 years old. I was in the kitchen, frantically answering the phone and getting dinner ready at the same time before their dad got home from work to tag-team parental duties with me, so I could race out the door, into rush-hour traffic, for a meeting across town. The girls were in the living room playing amiably, last I had checked. Despite my loud, hurried clattering in the kitchen, I could hear an argument brewing between them.

> "The purple ponies are *mine*," Sonja's tiny 2-year-old voice trailed into the kitchen.
> "I changed my mind. I want the purple one now," her big sister, Mia's, louder voice followed.

"Girls," I called from the kitchen, "there are more than enough ponies for both of you. You need to share, please." Repeat variations on this ineffective tactic numerous times over the course of endless minutes. Their bickering intensified as my attempts to distract and reprimand from the kitchen increased in volume, yet still went unheard. Before long, the girls went from amiable to hysterical, and I went from frustrated to furious. Dropping (or maybe I threw down) the spatula, I charged into the living room bellowing, "That is *enough*!" My hand was raised, my eyes were wide, my voice was loud enough to startle even me. It was a level of anger I didn't even know I could have. In the nanosecond before my up-raised hand descended on a little butt, I must have changed my mind. Instead of spanking, I grabbed a tiny wrist in each of my hands, dragged one daughter into their shared bedroom, the other into my bedroom, and slammed the doors.

Guilt and worry immediately swept in. I couldn't stop the mental interrogation that assaulted me, questioning my temperament, my parenting, my sense of control: What if I grabbed so hard I hurt my daughters? What if I'd left a bruise on their wrists? Would this spill over into other parts of my life? Could I get this angry at work? Could I lose my grip like that with anyone? Why did it materialize with my sweet little girls? What stopped me from carrying through with the intention of my upraised hand? Rather than feeling like I'd effectively handled the situation, I felt like the world's worst mother for not knowing how to deal with stress in the heat of a moment. My youngest daughter confirmed my anguish when she later told me I had turned into "Monster Mommy."

I spoke with my husband, Todd, that night. "I'm afraid of my anger," I told him. "Here I am, a 37-year-old social work professor with a PhD, loads of experience in this kind of thing, with few serious stressors in my life, but tonight, I nearly lost my shit and hit the small bodies of *our very own children.*" I was embarrassed and still shocked at what had happened. "My anger was so strong, I don't think I should spank the kids, it could be dangerous."

"I don't think I would ever spank our girls." He was already clear on his plans. He too had been spanked as a kid and watched his sister get spanked, by both their parents. But he was quite sure he would not spank our daughters. Strangely, we talk about everything in our lives, but we had never talked about spanking our kids.

As I talked with Todd, I realized that the last time I had physically hit someone was in 1986. I had punched him, my high school boyfriend (who later became my husband—surely that counts for something, right?), for some infraction I can no longer recall. I remember the basement family room we were in when I delivered the punch—in my parent's home; where I hit him—right in his gut; the shocked look on his face—he went from shocked to questioning. I don't even remember the reason why.

Why write and think so much about spanking? Because I want to know what spanking my kids would do not just to them but also to me. In one parenting book, readers are advised, "As a parent, you don't spank a child for your good; it is for the child's good." Still, I wonder about my good too. I wonder why we accept hitting children as a form of learning and discipline. I want to know why professionals, like social workers and pediatricians, rarely talk about it, and I want to know what all the research over the years can tell us. I became a social worker in the early 1990s, working with families who used physical punishment as part of their discipline practices, and with some families who outright abused their kids. I started wondering, where do we draw the line between a seemingly harmless, widely accepted discipline tactic and an abusive act with serious repercussions for both parent and child? Is there even a line?

I also began my parenting journey and was forced, along with my husband, to decide if we were going to spank. I can say that I grew up being spanked and turned out fine—many of us could say this. I'd already read dozens of parenting books. I was also a social work professor teaching students. I had researched parenting in public and how social spaces can encourage or discourage positive parenting. I taught international exchange students from countries where spanking is illegal and talked with them about their shock and dismay that spanking is legal in the United States. I had conversations with friends and family about spanking and witnessed good parents spank their kids. I scanned the research literature on spanking and learned it was robust and yet new to me. If I, as a social worker and professor, didn't know what the research findings on spanking were, I figured the average person certainly didn't. I found myself wanting to talk about spanking and realized that the research already existed; what we need is more conversation.

Nearly everyone knows what spanking is through personal experience. Most people alive today in the United States have delivered or received a spanking, or both. Even if you have never experienced one personally, you likely have a visceral understanding of the act. The majority of us believe that there are times when spanking is appropriate,[1] and many believe it is a loving and generous act of parenting when done right. We don't need research to tell us that most of us also believe that hurting children or teaching violence is never a good parental option. Despite that understanding, it seems we are polarized on the merit of spanking. The opinions we have are varied but are seldom informed beyond private experience.

The majority of families in the United States engage in some form of hitting, most of which is not tolerated: When siblings hit each other, it's called family fighting, and parents often intervene. When couples hit one another, it's called intimate partner violence, and the police get involved. When parents hit an adult child, or an adult child hits a parent, it is considered assault, a criminal act. Now, consider this: Parents hitting children on their buttocks is called spanking, whupping, paddling, or another benign label, and this is the only form of family hitting that not only is tolerated but also is legal, accepted, and often even encouraged.

My father was a Patternmaker working with complex, industrial, factory patterns. Translating a blueprint, he used wood or metal to create the first model of what would become a mass-produced product. He had large, rough hands and massive forearms that were monstrous to my child-sized eyes. He looked like Popeye, with his sleeves rolled up, exposing his bulging arms, and he often had a cigarette dangling from his mouth. There are five kids in my family, and according to discussions over the years, spanking was gendered in our 1970s household; my brothers report more spankings than my sister and me. But as a young girl, I distinctly remember the fear of being spanked by my father's strong hands.

One of my most vivid memories is when I was about five or six. I was a loud child, waltzing through the house one day singing *Oklahoma*—the whole damned musical!—at the top of my lungs. Not surprisingly, I woke my father from a nap. He stomped out of the bedroom and looked around menacingly to see who was making such a racket. I scrambled down the hallway in terror as he spied me and began to chase, bellowing at me to "Keep it quiet!"—and that is where the scene stops in my mind. I don't remember anymore. Is the memory gone because what happened after is so traumatic, that my body and brain won't let me remember? Or, did I not get spanked? I was the fifth child, a daughter. Did his age, his own experience, and my gender stop him from spanking me? I can't say with any certainty what the answer is.

My tiny mother, 5 feet, 1 inch and 120 pounds, struggled to spank any of us kids. It wasn't in her temperament. When she tried, it seemed like she was half-heartedly performing a duty she was expected to do but really wasn't that into. We thought it was more funny than scary. I remember my 8-year-old brother Andy, and myself at age 5, recklessly chasing each other around the living room, nearly toppling lamps and her Hummel collection, laughing and squealing as we played an indoor version of tag. My mom yelled at us from the kitchen to stop. Once, twice. There was no third time. She marched into the living room, grabbed Andy by the arm with one hand, and attempted to spank him with the other, but he out-wiggled her grip and ran across the room out of harm's reach. My mom spun around and, instead, came for me. I tried to wiggle loose too, but she held fast to my arm. Still, her flailing hits missed their target. My brother and I began to laugh. We knew we were already too old to be spanked, especially by such a small woman. She gave up and stormed back into the kitchen, throwing her standby threat, "Knock it off or it'll get worse!" over her shoulder like a wet dish towel.

A disciplinary technique my parents used on us when we fought with each other, that so resonated with me I intentionally chose to use with my children, was to force us to sit on the floor and look at each other. Just a foot or two away. No talking, no touching. Just sit and look one another in the eye. Those were the rules. This, too, is physical punishment—sitting, not moving, looking another person in the eye, forcing a body to experience something uncomfortable. The punishment, while not hitting, is still of the body, there is still a strong connection—perhaps even more so because we are forced to confront, eye to eye, the human in front of us, with whom we are in conflict. Ninety-nine percent of the time, we wound up giggling at each other.

We learn through the body, especially as children, when our brains are still developing and our complex thinking has not yet matured. The body holds the memory, the measurement of the feelings. Later, the mind explains the measurement, tallies the worthiness of what occurred, and gives it a story, usually one that includes being good or bad, but not one that includes complexity because we are a child. And so we explain the spankings we experienced, as unjust or deserved, or wretched or saving us, and the stories shape us.

I began to wonder, does a child think, *I am loved, that is why I am spanked. My parents care for my well-being and that is why I am spanked. They hope for my happiness, that is why I am spanked. Their love is so big, their dreams so high, their support so deep, that is why I am spanked.* That is what many believe because that is what we are told, and we don't question it. Historically, it's what some religions and experts have told us, what our parents, neighbors, and even strangers feel compelled to tell us. Just because so many people say something is true, does that make it true?

Even though the overwhelming majority of us have experienced spanking in our lives, we rarely talk about it publicly. Yet when I asked others about it, I was surprised that people had a lot to say. I think even they were surprised at how much. What I found is people often want to talk but may feel trepidation. Nearly everyone launched into their own private spanking story. Almost universally as the spankee. "Many a wooden spoon was broken over my behind!" "I was spanked, and it hurt, and I never did that again!" The facial expressions say more. Some people will quickly say that their spanking wasn't that harsh; others seem to not want to comment on severity. The story inside those short confessions is deeper and more complex. Ask these same adults if they spank their children, and the stories shift tone. Maybe they spanked one child, but that one needed it, or they gave their child a swat, not a spanking. Realistically, many of us have been a spanker, not just a spankee. Despite this commonality, a lot of us are not talking about it.

In the mid-1960s my parents received a handmade gift from my father's sister. Crafted from lightweight wood, the paddle is lovingly hand-painted by my Aunt Mary. Near the handle is a painted heart, followed by the words, "The Naughty Stick," in a calligraphic style, down the length of the paddle. At the other end of the paddle is a police officer with a whistle and bat. He's smirking but does not look menacing. Aunt Mary painted those images with family culture in mind. The Naughty Stick is about lovingly teaching kids through clear discipline. It hung, in a permanent spot, in my family home—where it could be easily grabbed by a parent. It seemed treacherous to face The Naughty Stick; luckily I have no memory of my parents ever hitting one of us with it. I recall the stick being waved by my parents in threat, or them smacking the palm of their hand in an angry warning to start doing the right thing. Over the years, the tales of family folklore have been recounted many times, and The Naughty Stick is a precious family heirloom.

Is spanking a problem? Historically, spanking has been viewed as an act that parents have the right and responsibility to do. Most families in the past evaluated spanking as good for children, as a useful tool to teach them how to behave, how to listen, how to control their impulses and get along in society. But meanings change over time, and what was once accepted or even ignored can become despised or condemned through new information, social trends, or value shifts.[2] While spanking used to be a childrearing question, it has now become a question of child protection and well-being[3] and, I believe, parental well-being.

If we have spanked our beloved children, we may feel vulnerable to share. The emotional exposure can feel overwhelming; unless we believe we have a really good reason to spank our child, then we may land in the world of justification and righteousness. The emotional vulnerability about disciplining our children can lead to strong feelings of control, fear, judgment, and a "manufacturing of certainty."[4] In some ways, it's human nature to want to deduce issues into categories of right or wrong, and then put people into these categories as we come across them. Against spanking? You're a permissive liberal who snowplows and helicopters their children into an easy life. For spanking? You're a narrow-minded autocrat with a short temper and not enough knowledge of parenting skills.

As a parent myself, the biggest challenge I found as I tried to determine whether I should spank my own kids was figuring out what it would do to me. I became a parent in my 30s, but I wasn't done growing and maturing. It seemed spanking my kids would fundamentally change me. Rationally, I know that most people who spank do not go around hitting other people. If they did, we would overwhelm our criminal justice system with charges of assault and battery. Still, I felt that if I spanked my kids, I was missing out on a chance to learn and grow myself—namely, could I do this parenting thing in a different, maybe more effective way, that doesn't involve hitting my children's bodies? Knowing how to process conflict, delicately balance complex negotiations, and fairly create boundaries with clear verbal authority, this is the stuff of modern parenting and modern citizenry. My dad once said to me, years before I ever had children, at a time when I was wondering if I even would, "I hope you have children someday. You'll learn so much about yourself." Hitting my kids didn't feel like a learning opportunity for *me*.

During these years reading, discussing, and thinking about spanking, I had a lot of memories of my own spankings and my four siblings' spankings. I also remember my parents' constant love for us. In the 1970s, my parents used to have dinner parties. The 1970s were a time when children didn't socialize in adult parties as they often do today. Shunned to the basement, I was supposed to entertain myself in the family room. But the open staircase beckoned. The distracted adults laughed and talked as the wine flowed. Creeping up the stairs and peering through the railings, I could watch and hear it all: My dad refreshing the drinks, clanking dinnerware, the appreciation of my mom's good cooking. And the talking, all the talking, so many voices swirling around, sharing benign gossip and funny stories, sometimes heartache or other sad news, politics, or religion. And most rare, yet most interesting to me, was when adults talked about their own struggle with something, a story of a mistake they made.

At 9 years old, I had a profound epiphany: Adults make mistakes too! Before that moment, I imagined only children made mistakes. That's why we were spanked and adults were not. I imagined a time of growing up when the problems of childhood would end. I would be all figured out. Instead, I eventually became an adult and found myself with more complex problems and an ever-developing sense of how to handle them, sometimes successfully, sometimes not. When I started writing this book at age 43, that time period of my imagined mistake-free adulthood had still not arrived. I am still waiting, still a growing person, peering through the railings, listening to stories, and marveling at the human experience. But it's now my job, as a social work professor.

This book began out of sincere interest in families—a captivation with family dynamics and how childhood and parenthood shape adult lives. A common belief is that good parenting bestows advantages for children and less-than-good parenting can have devastating consequences. I needed to know: Which side does spanking land on?

I first entered this issue of spanking believing the commonality of spanking made it benign. Spanking is nearly clandestine and yet everywhere. I was fascinated by the enormous amount of research on spanking that seemed overstudied and yet underdiscussed. I developed empathy for my parents who spanked me and empathy for parents who feel they must spank to keep their children safe or teach them an important lesson. Even empathy for parents who spank too much or too harshly. In my years of social work practice, I rarely, maybe never, met a family that truly wanted to hurt their child out of malice. Most families try their best to be loving, and like all humans, fail sometimes. Some of us fail harder or more frequently than others.

As an adult who was spanked and turned out fine, I started this project feeling open to a middle-of-the-road ending to this spanking debate. That waned. Study after study, story by story, I edged toward understanding that spanking should not be part of our modern world. By the end of this book, I found myself never believing a spanking is warranted—not just because it doesn't serve the child well but because it is no help for a parent either. Strangely, we hit the people we love the most. I now know that spanking is a form of family violence.

Hitting people smaller than us must have consequences—how could it not?

Acknowledgments

To the social scientists who produced decades of research on spanking. Many of them are referenced in this book. Thank you for your important work.

Dr. Christopher Cotten and Dr. Jacquelyn Vincson influenced the earliest version of this work. Thank you for your meaningful conversations. Melissa Sherlock, thank you for your keen eye and reading of early drafts, and your long-term dedication to children's well-being. Donald Gault shared invaluable guidance and feedback on the manuscript and held true to the recognition of parents as people too. His years of work in peaceful families and communities were guideposts in my thinking and writing. In the last stages of this book, Jennifer Hildebrandt, my writing coach, helped me write for people, not social scientists. Thank you.

Augsburg University, my academic home. Students, your classroom conversations helped me see there was more to talk about with this topic. The Undergraduate Research and Graduate Opportunity Office paid for a student researcher, Alexa Anderson, to research school spanking. Sadie Werlein, a social work student, completed an independent study on physical child abuse laws. The Center for Teaching and Learning at Augsburg University provided summer financial research and writing support. Thank you.

My partner Todd and our two daughters, Mia and Sonja, put up with my constant noting of spanking anywhere I saw it. I love and appreciate you more than you know. Thanks for letting me share parts of our family story.

I cannot thank my own family of origin more, especially my mom and dad. The experience of being spanked, watching my four siblings get spanked, and my Aunt Mary who made the Naughty Stick for our family were the original sources of inspiration for this book. Mom and Dad, you coupled those spankings with a never-ending font of love and support. I'm quite sure that's why I turned out fine.

PART I

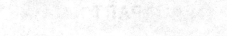

1

Whupping, Paddling, Smacking

A Spank by Any Other Name Still Stings

> "How shall we order the child?" is an age-old, often frantic question.
> When he misbehaves, shall we hit him, and, if so, how hard?[1]
>
> —Mary Cable

In September 2014, newspapers across the United States reported that Minnesota Vikings star running back Adrian Peterson had turned himself into police after a Texas grand jury indicted him on child injury charges. Peterson's 4-year-old son had shoved one of his siblings out from in front of a motorbike video game console. As a punishment, Peterson had stripped a switch from a tree, removed all the leaves, and whipped the child with it, leaving cuts and bruises on the boy's back, buttocks, ankles, legs, and scrotum.

The shocking details of the case elicited harsh criticism, most of it leveled at Peterson. It also provoked—or resuscitated—a national debate about physical punishment. Sportscasters, journalists, commentators, childcare experts, and even fellow athletes weighed in. On the topic of spanking, everyone was an expert. In one opinion piece, CNN commentator Mel Robbins states: "[H]it a 4-year-old and you can call yourself a 'loving father'? That's completely screwed up."[2] Dr. Jared Pingleton, a psychologist and minister, railed in his *Time* published op-ed piece that "there is a giant chasm between a mild spanking properly administered out of love and an out of control adult venting their emotions by physically abusing a child."[3] The NFL's decision to suspend Peterson for 15 games was alternately condemned for being too lenient and too severe.

Peterson maintained that he had never intended to hurt his son and professed that much of the criticism leveled against him was rooted in cultural misunderstanding. In fact, he went further by declaring that he would not be the success he is today were it not for the "whuppings" he received from his own father. Peterson stated, "I am not a perfect parent, but I am, without a

Spanked. Christina L. Erickson, Oxford University Press. © Oxford University Press 2022.
DOI: 10.1093/oso/9780197518236.003.0001

doubt, not a child abuser."[4] In 2018, Peterson reiterated his commitment to whupping as a disciplinary tactic he frequents as needed, especially for repeat offenses. While he does use other modes of discipline, he declared, "[I] didn't let the previous incident change me."[5]

The fact that a case like Peterson's was able to stir such a range of public reactions illustrates America's mixed feelings regarding physical punishment. And whether you call it spank, smack, whup, paddle, or pop, everyone seems to have an opinion.

"All those kids carrying Uzis on the street? Their mothers hit the hell out of them," proclaimed Oprah Winfrey on an episode about spanking during her television show's heyday.[6] The talk show, which ran from 1986 to 2011, offered an entire episode on spanking in May 1994. In it, Winfrey introduces us to Kim and Marcus McDaniel, a couple who look to the Bible for guidance on childrearing and view spanking as "loving discipline." Says Kim, "When God chooses to give you children—the instant that child is born into this world—you are the delegated authority over those children at that point."

Kim and Marcus allow a camera crew into their home to film them with their two young daughters. "This is the instrument that we use," says Kim, holding up a wooden dowel, about 16 inches in length. "It does the job: it stings, it hurts." She whacks herself on her bare thigh. "I mean, you can just do it to your leg and it hurts. We tried it out. . . . It'll make a mark." The camera cuts to the youngest daughter sitting on the floor, mid-tantrum. Kim, squatting beside her, rises to get the stick. We hear the slap of the stick on the little girl's thigh and the child's scream while Kim says, "Look at my face. Look at my face. Daddy told you when you can have some juice. Look at me. You may have juice in a few minutes." The toddler continues shrieking, and Kim administers another whack: "You stop."

The McDaniels, who keep another stick in their car, tell Oprah's audience that after a spanking is one of the most special times between a parent and child: "You have an opportunity to love your child," says Kim. "We do not use our hands to hit our children. Your hands are to love your children." Winfrey, one of America's most visible survivors of child maltreatment, is unable to feign neutrality. She challenges an audience member who is defiantly defending spanking: "My question to you is simply this: Aren't children just little people with feelings just like big people have? And don't they feel the same kind of humiliation, degradation, embarrassment when they are slapped in public as you would feel? Don't they feel the same thing?" Kim McDaniel is reassuring. "Children are real forgiving; they are," she states. "If they weren't, they'd hate us."

Indeed, not unlike Adrian Peterson, many adults spanked as children defend its practice as effective.[7] When another guest on Winfrey's panel is asked whether the harsh spankings helped her, she replies "yes" before qualifying her answer: "to a degree." A beating, she says, was the only way to get through to her as a child. And isn't the proof in the pudding? She has grown into a poised and successful adult. Winfrey is unconvinced. "It doesn't matter what a person has accomplished in life or how many things they have attained," she asserts. Having "made it" doesn't justify spanking in Winfrey's eyes. But proponents of spanking still say that if done right, a loving parent disciplines well to include spanking.

"The general rule for spanking is this: it needs to be done at the right TIME, in the right WAY, in the right PLACE and for the right REASONS," says Bishop Dave Chikosi, of Nehandra Radio.[8] With all those requirements, no wonder it's difficult to determine when and if it's right to spank a child.

Spanking Defined

The word corporal, meaning "of or belonging to the body," is derived from the Latin word *corporalis*: the body. One of the earliest references to "corporal punishment"—punishment of the body—appeared more than 400 years ago, in the 1580s.[9] The word spank, "to strike forcefully with the open hand, especially on the buttocks," began as a verb and can be traced back to 1727; it is thought to perhaps have been imitative of the sound that results. It took another 50-plus years to show up as a noun.[10] The word whup appeared in the late 19th century as a variant of "whip."[11] The words we have chosen over the years affect our sensibilities on the acceptability of a hitting. Whipping and flogging were common terms before 1930, but those terms used today would be shocking. Popping, swatting, whupping, and spanking are the acceptable terms used in our current society. Depending on your geographic location, setting, or culture, spanking, whupping, popping, smacking, and paddling are terms that are often conflated to mean the same thing—a hit to the buttocks to cause pain, with the intent to discipline or teach a lesson. From this point on, I'll use the more common term *spanking*, for clarity, unless otherwise indicated.

Spanking is the most common term for hitting a child on the behind, followed by swat, and both are generally considered acceptable.[12] This acceptable terminology normalizes and veils what is really happening. The words conceal very different experiences for the person being hit and the hitter. The term dampens the sharpness of that reality: A big person hitting a smaller person. Even though spanking is hitting a part of the body, it is the only hitting considered a form of discipline, rather than a form of violence.[13] How do our language and labels support our acceptance and use of certain behaviors? If spanking is never considered hitting or a form of violence, it will likely always be accepted. Spanking acceptance is also partly due to where spankings are given—the butt. The butt is the least dangerous place to hit someone. There are no vulnerable organs, it is a meatier section of the body, and hitting it risks less serious injury. Importantly, bruises and welts are covered by clothing, ensuring the secrecy of the hitting. Our norming spanking as acceptable is supported by benign terms and veiled body parts and by the words we don't use: hitting and violence.

Spanking is generally considered the open hand on the buttocks, but we know that the variations on spanking are numerous, from a covered to bare bottom, to using an implement like a kitchen spoon or shoe to a switch taken from a tree. Also consider velocity, strength of the spanker, number of hits, age or size of the child, and parent's temperament, and the variations are endless.

Who Spanks?

The General Social Survey (GSS) is a long-running research project surveying US citizens to discern changing attitudes and norms over decades. The survey is conducted by the nonpartisan and objective research organization, NORC, at the University of Chicago and is funded by the National Science Foundation. The GSS is a highly regarded research endeavor and is considered the best measure of attitudinal trend data in the United States. The survey covers a range of questions, from straightforward and simple questions such as "how happy are you?" to more complex and potentially conflictual questions such as acceptance of marijuana use, sexual activities, and attitudes toward civil liberties. Because every household in the United States has an equal chance of being surveyed, and the questions have now been asked over decades, the responses can capture largely accepted trends over time. Since 1986, they have been asking this question: "Do you strongly agree, agree, disagree, or strongly disagree that it is sometimes necessary to discipline a child with a good, hard spanking?" Since that first survey, the responses to this question have ranged from 65% to nearly 90% of responders strongly agreeing or agreeing with that statement.[14] When the question was first asked in 1986, 83% of respondents agreed with it. In 2000, 73% of respondents agreed, and the most recent data available from the GSS, from 2018, indicated that 66% of respondents agreed with the statement. So, although a majority of people in the United States believe in spanking, the trend appears to be heading slowly downward.

Other research suggests that more parents spank, and likely more often, than the GSS reveals. Perceived cultural approval of spanking is a strong predictor of whether parents use the technique, despite what they personally believe.[15] Disbelief in spanking does not manifest in the scenarios of home life. The broad cultural acceptance of spanking is so indelibly linked to parenting that even parents who don't believe in spanking have used it at times when their child has been the most misbehaved. They may not consider themselves a spanking family, but at the moment that the act of perceived misbehavior occurred, in the privacy of the family home, it was believed to be warranted. As one parent I spoke with rationalized, "I don't spank my kid but I did have to swat him on the butt a few times." Spanking is a deeply held belief, constant through generations, that confirms that in certain circumstances, a child deserves it, no questions asked, no need to explain. "The cultural norm that says parents are morally obligated to hit children 'when necessary' is probably the most fundamental reason why so many children are hit."[16]

In general, the justifying scenario goes like this: A parent has told a child to stop misbehaving, possibly multiple times, yet the child continues. Or the child has gotten "too big for their britches" and needs to know in no uncertain terms who the parent is. Or the child has done something dangerous that seems to warrant a spanking even before a verbal reprimand, such as running into the street. In these circumstances, many people have hit one or more of their children, one or more times.

Those who admit to spanking are likely to underestimate the amount of times they use it for discipline. Parents' memory of how often they spanked their children is lower than when audiotapes and videotapes are in the home and capture the actual number of spankings given.[17] Either they don't remember because it is a common enough activity to be nonmemorable, or they feel a spanking stigma and wish to present themselves more favorably. Either way, the privacy of the family home, combined with the consistent majority of US citizens who respond positively to the GSS and the normed acceptance of spanking, indicates that most parents in the United States spank. And many do around the world too. Because most of us were spanked, most of us grow up to spank our children. Experiencing spanking as a child, especially if it wasn't overly harsh or excessively frequent, encourages us to repeat it.[18] And so, spanking continues.

Over the years researchers have delved into data to find out who spanks more. Efforts to determine whether some groups of people spank more than others have come up muddled. In one 2-week study of college-educated mothers, some never spanked and others spanked nine times per week.[19] Hispanic parents born and raised in the United States tend to spank more than Hispanic parents born in other countries.[20] Teen moms are more likely to utilize spanking.[21] The poorer the family, the more likely they are to spank.[22] The more children a family has, the more likely the family is to spank.[23] Women who became mothers unexpectedly found that they spanked their children more frequently.[24] Regionally, people who live in the Northeast corner of the United States spank the least, and those in the Southeast states spank the most.[25]

Overall, moms tend to spank more, found in repeated studies, even when that was not the question of interest. Moms are even more likely to spank if they have additional elder caregiver duties.[26] Mothers who reported that they had more childcare duties than they could handle often used physical punishment and spanking more frequently than mothers who did not feel overburdened with childcare duties.[27] Long hours of parenting can be stressful, and it seems plausible that more time spent with kids could run patience dry. Marital conflict and family stress, in their many forms, increase spanking frequency.[28] Depressive symptoms in parents,[29] especially dads, are linked to spanking, and single mothers who begin a serious relationship are more likely to spank.[30] But moms who work tend to spank less, even if they experience depression.[31]

Caveats

The *but* here is pretty big—if you dig deep enough into the research findings, you are almost sure to find a study that disputes the findings just identified. They may be in small caveats, or not a major finding, but contradictory findings on who spanks more are seen over and over again. While large-scale demographics influence our spanking practices, our family experiences, and our beliefs about children and adults, authority, morals, and even what we consider "naughty" play a part. Not surprisingly, parents who believe in spanking and have positive attitudes about spanking tend to be the most consistent spankers.[32] Parents who spank most frequently believe in spanking's effectiveness, expect a positive outcome from the spanking, and have little guilt about the discipline. Parents who feel guilty after spanking their child tend to spank less.[33] The more meaningful differences in spanking are related to intensity, frequency, and paired behavior with the spanking, such as yelling or name-calling.

So we turn again to the GSS and the trend of spanking data over more than 30 years as our most reliable indicator of who spanks. The GSS does categorize data on some cross-cutting variables. Seventy-seven percent of Black people, 64% of White people and 63% of "others" (that's how respondents are classified in the data) agreed with spanking in 2018.[34] That means that the majority of all people, across racial identities, believe children sometimes need a good hard spanking.

One universal instigator of spanking any family could experience is economic hardship. Over the decades of the GSS, people with lower economic attainment had a higher acceptance of spanking, and these trends have held steady over time. In 2018, 76% of parents in the lowest socioeconomic group (self-described) agreed with the spanking question, while 48% of those describing themselves in the highest socioeconomic group agreed with spanking.[35] In smaller studies across the decades, the support for spanking and the valuing of unquestioning obedience is higher among people with lower financial attainment.[36]

Economic factors affecting spanking have several explanations. One common belief is that a person's responsiveness to authority, learned in childhood through obedience to parents, is key to attaining success in employment as an adult.[37] Working-class families may expect unquestioning obedience from their children, with physical threats a foundation to enforce this obedience, while middle- and upper-class families have freedoms to allow more self-direction.[38] Years of formal education can intersect with income too, suggesting that income and education can promote a sense of ability to handle difficulties without force or promote access to other options.[39] Parents in lower income communities have fewer material resources to use in controlling their children; physical punishment is a cheap and readily available option for parents with few privileges to take away and little money for enticing rewards.[40] Having a lot of advantages or privileges can allow parents a sense of relief from authoritarianism and physical punishment. Economic stress influences adults' patience and sense of time. Parents struggling to make ends meet may not have the emotional bandwidth for long conversations and need quick behavioral change from their children. Children behaving well at home, even if through force, can bring a sense of stability when economic hardship causes instability.[41]

Families that have moved up the economic ladder after coming from a financially disadvantaged background often continue to hold onto the belief in spanking as an important parental duty. Some families have been found to approve of more authoritarian methods of discipline, including spanking, across their income level.[42] Having a financially disadvantaged background is related to parental support of authoritarian childrearing,[43] often manifested in the use of spanking. For many families this is a response to harsh and unwelcoming social conditions, as well as outright danger experienced by poor people and people of color in the United States, even from entities meant to serve them, such as schools, police, and social service institutions. Privilege allows more room for mistakes.

Times of economic recession increase the use of spanking. In the 2008 economic recession, "high-frequency spanking" (identified in this study as spanking that happens at least 11 times a year) rose with each drop in percent of consumer confidence. Consumer confidence is a strong indicator of the well-being of the larger economy; fear and insecurity can rise as consumer confidence decreases, increasing stress and the possibility of harsh discipline from parents. High-frequency spankers are more than three times as likely to be contacted by Child Protective Services. The people who had the largest increase in spanking during the 2008 recession were mothers with higher educational levels and income.[44] Clearly, what is happening in the wider world does affect our parenting and how we discipline. Fears and anxieties resulting from economic recessions, pandemics, climate change, elections, and even their own work struggles are enough to put parents on edge and increase their choice to spank rather than employ another discipline tactic. These recession findings suggest that the stress of economic factors likely influence spanking even more than the category of one's income.[45]

All of this is to say that there's an inherent problem in trying to pin spanking on specific groups of people. It shields us from the larger social context and macro forces that shape family behavior. It also ignores the findings of the GSS, arguably a far more valid and reliable measure than any other study, which continuously shows that most people in the United States believe in "a good hard spanking," at least sometimes. While reported acceptance of spanking is trending downward, younger generations are still in favor. The *Washington Post* claimed that Millennials are not changing the status: "Support for spanking children has been mostly locked in place for three decades and appears here to stay."[46]

For every group of people, some believe in spanking some of the time. Understanding who spanks more is interesting, but that research had its time and place. Modern families don't always separate along specific economic, religious, or racial lines anymore. We intermarry and co-parent along every line of human diversity imaginable. We move and are mobile on a global level. Most worrisome is that identifying spankers makes us think we are somehow different from them, rather than recognizing they are us. Pinpointing who spanks may cause us to look at other people with suspicion and wonder about their spanking practices, rather than reflect on our own family dynamics.

Who Gets Spanked?

Most kids get spanked. Five percent of parents report spanking by 3 months of age and 8 percent by 8 months of age.[47] Spanking most frequently begins at about age 1 year, rising in frequency until age 3, which is the peak of spanking,[48] with a slow decline up through the teen years when spanking becomes far less common. Like the tails in a bell curve, there are people who spank before age 1 and after age 12, but the percentages are smaller. Take Liz, for example, a new parent in her late 20s, busy attending graduate school and working part-time. She was married, bright, caring, and happy to be a parent for the first time. She was frustrated and perplexed though. Liz's 11-month-old daughter was not cooperating during bath time. She would refuse to sit in her little tubby, force her legs as straight as she could, standing and wailing while her mom, bent over the tub, attempted to bathe her. Coaxing didn't work; distraction and play failed. Exasperated, she felt the only way the little girl would learn to sit in the tub was to spank her. Liz had no way of knowing why she wouldn't sit down. The water was warm but not hot, she held her to feel safe; it just seemed the baby was fighting it out of obstinance. So she spanked her and still felt perplexed.

Boys, after age 2, are spanked more often, in study after study, from Hong Kong to Ireland, and lots of places in between.[49] Many children in modern society attend preschool or daycare, which means outsourcing parenting chores can provide a break from family duties. Less time with parents means less time spanked. Preschool participation is related to fewer spankings.[50] Children who are more difficult, or at least perceived to be that way, elicit harsher parenting practices, including spanking, from their parents, and this has been confirmed over many studies.[51] A temperamental or challenging child can trigger parents to use a method of discipline they may not even want to use. Younger mothers who report that their child is difficult, experience stress, and espouse fewer alternatives to physical punishment are more likely to spank their child.[52] We spank when frustrated.[53] We spank less when the fathers are supportive, even prenatally supportive.[54] Spankings are twice as likely to happen in the evening than they are at any other time of day. The easiest explanation for this is fatigue and hunger.[55] Hunger causes kids to be cranky and parents to feel short-fused. Kids whose parents are concerned about their development or behavior are spanked and yelled at more.[56] People are more likely to spank if they live in a community in which spanking is normalized, meaning lots of families spank their kids and other people know.[57]

Spanking can occur anytime in childhood up until age 18, when the child reaches full legal adulthood. At the age of 18, spanking your child becomes assault.

Assumptions

The act of spanking a child, for most parents, is rooted in their own experiences growing up. The adage that "I got spanked and I turned out fine" is an oft-told rationale to support the practice. Discipline causes more uncertainty than any other time in parenting. In those flashpoints when discipline is necessary, we expect parents to have considered research from experts, folk wisdom from family members, and advice from peers, and in that quagmire of parental angst, to discipline their child with certainty. When the moment spanking becomes a potential parenting tool—usually early in the toddler years—we often have unexamined assumptions and tools from the last generation that emerge from a moment of stress. Like all people, we move to what we know best: our own experiences. Most of the time it has worked, more or less. Many more of us are spanked than not spanked. While there is violence in our society, there are also great resources of love and kindness—most created by people who were spanked.

These assumptions underlie a few demanding and, frankly, sometimes scary, facts. Spanking has been associated with poor school outcomes, aggression, crime, struggles with mental health, intimate partner violence, and even lower lifetime incomes. So do parents have all the information available? Since the 1950s, studies have shown a relationship between aggressive behavior and spanking.[58] Spanking research has a long and robust history in disciplines such as psychology and sociology. How available this information has been to the average citizen is questionable. At the same time, we expect parents to take their parenting job seriously. Few things can rouse the frustration of people more than a parent who appears to be lazy or disinterested— the parent who just doesn't take a stance, for whom the children seem to be raising themselves. Loving parents are expected to do so actively—and they teach their kids with intention. The assumption that spanking is a tool in a loving parent's toolbox is a powerful script, and one we have turned to for generations. The trick is, some of our assumptions are insidious, and we may not even know where they came from. Sociologist Dr. Murray Straus claimed that spanking assumptions had roots in seeing children as potentially evil.[59]

"Beating the devil out of them" was the underlying assumption of spanking. Whupping children has been associated with the "cradle to prison pipeline" for families. Are we aware of the fuller meaning of our assumptions and how they influence our choices today? Has anyone ever asked what spanking does to the parents? The research on spanking is robust, yet our assumptions rarely match the research.

While spanking is a physical act, it is really a form of communication. We may think we are spanking to teach a lesson about running out in a busy street, showing too much "attitude," or fighting with siblings, though we are as likely to communicate much more about who is worthy and important, our place in the world, what is valued and how authority and power work. Sometimes spankings are a parental response to activities that occurred well before the spanking even happened. Stress at work could be one culprit. Many of us remember the spanking but not what we were spanked for. Does the lesson stick? What can likely resonate with a lot of us is that the effects of spanking differ from family to family and from culture to culture.[60] Spanking in one family may be used as an assertion of parental authority, or an initial attention-grabber followed by additional consequences, while in others it may be used as an act of aggression. There are a lot of ways to spank a child. The growing fear of "your father coming home," the quick swat, the spanking in anger, to get the child's attention, to really hurt and make someone remember, the open hand or the belt, stick, paddle, cord, the private whupping, and the public paddling. Spanking is about so much more than the hit itself.

Spanking is considered a loving act by some and a short slide to abuse by others. It is private and emotional, but it has legal standing too. Spanking one's children is legal in all 50 states and in many of the 197 countries worldwide. While child abuse is not legal anywhere in the United States, parents have the right to determine the best ways to discipline and teach their children, and that does include hitting them. The strong belief that spanking is a necessary disciplinary act is undergirded by the 19 states that allow paddling in school as a form of discipline.[61] Grandparents, nannies, and other caregiving adults may spank when they are in charge of taking care of the kids—sometimes. Parents have the right to teach their children as they wish, including allowing others to discipline them, so long as they don't jeopardize their health, fail to educate them, or abuse them physically or emotionally. If that happens, people expect caring professionals to step in, such as teachers, nurses, social workers, and faith leaders. But how do we know what's the right amount of spanking and what's not? The devil is in the details, and the details are worth exploring.

2
History and Mystery

> The history of childhood is a nightmare from which we have only re-
> cently begun to awaken.[1]
>
> —L. DeMause

In our oldest record, including medieval times, the concept of childhood didn't exist.[2] Childhood developed over time, influenced by economic changes, elongating life spans, and advances in knowledge. It was not until the 17th century that the idea of children as anything other than mini adults was accepted. Childhood is a construct of only the past few hundred years, and human reckoning of how our earliest years set up the trajectory of the rest of our lives is still forming. Building on our knowledge of brain develop-ment, and social and emotional health, societies around the world have ex-tended the length of childhood and called for recognition of this special time in human development. Humans didn't start out that way.

Indeed, birth and early childhood were challenging times even just a few hundred years ago. Extreme forms of child maltreatment included infanti-cide, servitude, limited nutrition, forced work in small spaces, and physical punishment that was tantamount to torture.[3] Parents, teachers, and ministers alike believed that the only cure for childhood foolishness was by spanking with a rod or whip. It was accepted, even supported by law, that parents and parental proxies such as ministers and teachers[4] had the right to determine appropriateness and intensity of physical punishments.

This historical record is limited by its Eurocentric recording. Much of our recorded history is based on colonizers' writings, or in languages, such as English, that dominate the research landscape today. It is, by default, the his-tory of people with economic power at that time and with access to contribute to the written word. Indeed, some nations believe that whipping and spanking of children were an outcome of European colonization of their land and cul-ture.[5] Much of the history of childhood is a sad reprise of disparities across skin color and gender, including rates of poverty, access to primary school,

Spanked. Christina L. Erickson, Oxford University Press. © Oxford University Press 2022.
DOI: 10.1093/oso/9780197518236.003.0002

and childhood labor. What we do know is that European historians found that "the further back one goes in history, the less effective parents are in meeting the developmental needs of the child."[6]

As far as we know, parents have always physically punished their children. Much of the history of children is a story of punishment, dealing with adversity, and starting adulthood early. Because spanking has been considered a prerogative of parents and a normal aspect of daily life, it was not often considered worthy of record keeping,[7] and there are historical gaps in which no one wrote about it. What we do know is that since humanity began, childhood has elongated, opportunities for children have broadened, and types of physical punishment have narrowed.

1600 to 1800

A dominant method of childrearing for discipline and learning in both Europe and the colonial United States was harsh physical punishment including isolation, beatings, and withholding meals.[8] During the 15th to 17th centuries, severe physical punishment was frequent. The thin branch of a birch tree was the implement of choice in Europe and was imported to the United States and called a switch.[9] The literature of the period, such as Eleazar Moody's 1634 *School of Good Manners*, described the petty "offenses" that could be characterized as "stubborn" and worthy of punishment: not bowing when passing one's parent, going outdoors without permission, or sullenness for parental mandates. There was believed to be a "stubbornness of mind" that had to be broken down in children for them to learn obedience, and this created "severe and arbitrary modes of discipline in Colonial days."[10]

During these years there was little question that parents had the right, even duty, to beat their offspring. In colonial Massachusetts, the "Stubborn Child Law," inspired by biblical injunctions in the book of Deuteronomy (21:20-21),[3] allowed children to be beaten or even put to death for obstinate behavior. The law, passed in 1646, stated:

> If a man have a rebellious or stubborn son of sufficient years of understanding, viz., sixteen, which will not obey the voice of his father or the voice of his mother, and that when they have chastened him will not harken unto them. . . . Such a son shall be put to death.[11]

Similar statutes were passed in Connecticut in 1650, Rhode Island in 1668, and New Hampshire in 1679.[12] Parenting in this period focused on inborn sin and techniques to assure children's evil inclinations could be snuffed out or at least formed into decency.[13] Any methods to do so were supported. As quoted by a philosopher in 1748:

> It is quite natural for the child's soul to want to have a will of its own, and things that are not done correctly in the first two years will be difficult to rectify thereafter. One of the advantages of these early years is that force and compulsion can be used. Over the years, children forget everything that happened to them in early childhood. If their wills can be broken at this time, they will never remember afterwards that they had a will, and for this very reason the severity that is required will not have any serious consequence.[14]

Alternative views did emerge with some support. Educational advocate John Locke wrote in 1692 in *Some Thoughts on Education*:

> I would have children very seldom beaten. Tis to make slaves and not virtuous men to use them to be governed by the fear of the scourge and to know no other motive of their actions, no other rule of right and wrong, but the cudgel. . . . A gentle persuasion and reasoning will most times do much better. You will perhaps wonder to find me mention reasoning with children, and yet I cannot but think that the true way of dealing with them. They understand it as early as they do language, and if I misobserve not they love to be treated as rational creatures sooner than is imagined.[15]

Locke's ideas were slow to influence educational systems and even slower to reach the privacy of the home.[16]

1800 to 1900

The idea that a child's will must be broken, and done so before bad behavior took hold, continued as a common perception of good parenting. *A Mother's Magazine*, a periodical written in 1843 from the Calvinist, Christian point of view, described the frustration of parents of a 16-month-old girl who refused to say, "Dear Mama" when ordered by her father. When a 10-minute isolation in a room alone did not convince her, she was whipped and asked again. It took 4 hours, but the child finally obeyed. The mother reported in the magazine that the little girl was now always submissive to the will of her parents.[17] In the late 1800s, it is estimated that 100% of children received corporal punishment with a tool such as a whip or a stick.[18]

An event in 1829, widely reported in newspapers that engendered public outcry, is considered one of the early turning points for which people began "a gentling attitude toward children."[19] The story was self-told by a minister regarding the child he brought into his home to raise, a widow's son. One morning, during a lesson on spelling, the 4-year-old boy was requested to spell the word "gutter." The minister was sure the boy knew how to spell it but refused to do so out of willful contrariness. He threatened to whip the boy, and when the boy continued to refuse to spell the word, he took the boy to the cellar, stripped him, and beat him with birch tops, following the quote from the Christian Bible, "thou shalt beat him with the rod, and shalt deliver his soul from hell." The minister, fearing disobedient children, stated that it was better to break the child's will than to break his own word. The birch sticks eventually gave out, and when the child still could not spell the word, he garnered another stick and continued the whipping until the child was subdued. At this point, he described the child as "unusually mild, submissive, pleasant and interesting." He reported that the child ate a good dinner, and said, "I never had anybody so kind to me as you are." The child died a few days later. The outcry that ensued signaled a budding recognition of the harm of severe physical punishment.[20]

In 1847, Lyman Cobb, the author of *Evil Tendencies of Corporal Punishment as a Mean of Moral Discipline in Families and Schools, Examined and Discussed*, stated his love for children was the impetus for the book, and his knowledge came from being in classrooms in which some teachers taught with kindness and others with flogging. Cobb begins with a litany of biblical passages that have been used to support hitting children and contradicts them with biblical passages clearly against such punishment. Arguing that the moral upbringing of children is of the highest precedence, Cobb states that physical punishment "is more productive of evil than good results."[21] Cobb's book lays out 30 distinct objections to the use of the rod for hitting children. For example, Cobb notes, hitting is often done in haste and without thought; there are often injuries to the child; and it destroys joy between parent or teacher and the child. He then lays out 40 ways to prevent or substitute the use of the rod, including that parents and teachers should build patience, speak with kindness, and recognize their own erring ways. Dozens of letters and resolutions from influential people and groups are included in the appendices of Cobb's book, supporting his treatise on ending the use of the rod in hitting children.

Children's history scholars note that parenting during this time was authoritarian, and advice given about parenting had no hesitation or suggestion but rather represented directives for parents to follow for all children, without alternatives.[22] Most of the self-appointed child experts of the time backed up their advice in scripture.[23] As scholars note, perhaps what is clear is that "breaking" the will of children did produce people who followed rules and standards, but it did not generate peaceful people. Instead, it created people who felt comfortable with this kind of conflict.[24] Before 1860, most letters, books, newspapers, and magazines on parenting advice were written with total authority. People believed they had the right answers to parenting dilemmas and that parents should follow them without hesitation. Children were seen homogeneously, without uniqueness, so much so that only one method of discipline was needed.

From 1860 to the First World War, harsh physical punishment waned.[25] In the late 1800s a shift toward more nurturing approaches grew in family life, alongside the suffragists' movement for women and the ending of slavery. Some say it reflected an emphasis on maternal influence on children's lives over traditional authoritarian discipline driven by fathers. [26] People began to have more empathy for children, and the recognition of childhood as a unique time of life emerged. As the rod and whip declined, the hand gained popularity, and "spanking" earned acceptance and support as a typical family disciplinary practice, widely used by all parents, and considered much more humane than the whips and rods of previous years.

Another early effort to publicly question physical punishment inside the family home can be traced to an 1884 periodical, *The Ladies Home Journal*. In this first year of publication, it ran an article titled "Hasty Mothers," stating that whipping is not required to make children obedient.[27] In subsequent issues the column suggested that whipping can crush a child's independence, destroy a sense of moral relationship between the parent and child, and even awaken "animal instincts."[28] Other articles in the periodical advocated for children being allowed to determine their own adult lives and recognizing innate goodness, rather than depravity. As the century turned, these new parenting ideas continued to grow, broadening in acceptance.

1900 to 1920

In the early 1900s, as the industrial era was ushered in, many people lost their crafts, small businesses, and farms and became part of a mass of faceless laborers in large factories. Families felt not only the increase in economic pressures but also the loss of dignity and respect that came with the loss of their trade or talents. As a consequence, dejected parents felt the need to exert power and demand respect from someone, and that someone was often their children.[29] In these times of economic disparity, parents at the bottom of the economic hierarchy with limited social power to garner respect and compliance from their children used spanking to demand adherence to family rules and values.

In the big cities of the East Coast, children without adult supervision were a common sight; parents were often laborers working long hours, and public school was not yet a norm. Children roamed the streets in packs, from as young as 5, without a parent's watchful eye. Kids were lured outside because of the discomforts of the cramped quarters they lived in. The streets of Boston and New York were fraught with potential problems, crime, and victimization for children, causing fear and anxiety in already overburdened parents. In response, parents often used physical discipline, a desperate yet seemingly quick way to teach their children to avoid danger and trouble.[30]

Seeing the struggles of families in these large urban cores, the early 1900s ushered in an age of increased concerns regarding the rights of children, especially by a new class of "child savers." The child-saving movement was largely driven by white middle- and upper-class women with time for philanthropic endeavors. Driven by fears of the fate of immigrant children in urban areas, child savers waged campaigns aimed at making the public aware that children were not simply little adults. Among the movement's accomplishments were child labor laws, public education, and the nation's first court for juveniles.[31] These movements set the stage for society to view children differently, and opposition to the typical demands of complete obedience or physical punishment began to grow. A new idea emerged. "Training" a child could be as effective as a whipping, and encouragement could work as well as demands.[32]

1920 to 1950

Shifting ideas of parents' roles in the lives of children, as well as a beginning understanding of the longer term influence of parenting, was building. "No children should be brought up to fear their parents," stated the President of the Royal Medico-Psychological Society in 1929, claiming that maladjusted adults were the victims of parental mismanagement.[33] In response to this idea that parents influence their children's lives over the long term, the first formal parenting groups in the United States were offered by the Child Study Association of America, led by early social workers and nurses. Child Study Groups were described as "a gathering of parents who meet together for the purpose of learning about the best ways to bring up their children."[34] The most requested topic was disciplinary problems,[35] including how to make children behave "without so much whipping." Asked about their assessment of a group in Harlem, a leader wrote that a mother replied, "[D]oes less whipping, yet gets better results. Has saved herself from getting all worked up and just almost ready to explode sometimes and that seems to help more than anything else."[36] The idea of parent training, rather than only child training, had begun. As modern child welfare services began to form, one of it's advocates, Howard Hopkirk, demanded in 1929, "It is time we were putting the orphan asylums, with the stocks and whipping posts, in the background of a rejected heathenism."[37] In 1930, Howard Hopkirk presented an idea in a presentation he titled, "The Problem Child or the Child With a Problem," suggesting a turn toward respect for children as people with problems, not the problem itself.

In 1930, the *Journal of Education* signaled a transformation with their clearly titled article, *Stop Whipping Children* by Alice Park. She believed that size is the reason adults whip children, the proof being that whipping ends as soon as the child is large enough to strike back. Park identified the unseen effects of a whipping: "Feelings of bitterness, hatred, and even revenge rankle in the heart of the child."[38] Park claimed the destruction of a child's self-respect is the worst outcome of all.[39] Questions about hitting children raised practical concerns, like, does it work? Is there harm? The Child Study Association of America noted that authority maintained by fear is very short-lived, and the first inclination that physical punishment may be a source of bad behavior was considered, "It may lead to untruthfulness and other deception."[40] These kinds of questions began to slowly put to bed the idea that parents must hit children to make them obey.

In 1938, a mother who wrote to a newspaper advice column regarding her third-grade daughter's issues with mathematics was scolded for even thinking about physical punishment. "Would you give her a sound spanking or use other means to correct her trouble?" asked the mother. The reply from the columnist, child psychologist Dr. Garry Cleveland Myers, who later founded the children's magazine *Highlights*, a staple in the waiting rooms of countless pediatricians' offices, was unequivocal: "Please do not spank that child for her troubles with arithmetic or any other learning difficulties. Don't even look or breathe as if angry at her errors. Discipline yourself to be calm and patient. Otherwise, keep away from her while she tries to learn." He even infers that the mother herself may be the cause of the academic problems: "Her trouble is not carelessness but emotional confusion."[41]

These new views on hitting and children's development were beginning to reach the masses, albeit without full acceptance. A general shift from thinking of children as "economically worthless" to "emotionally priceless" was slowly growing.[42] Angelo Patri was an Italian American author and educator who had a decades-long syndicated newspaper column, *Our Children*, and hosted a

weekly radio show from 1928 to 1943. Spanking was a regular topic. His newspaper columns clearly rejected the practice of spanking, as did most of his
personalized replies to parents who wrote to him. Patri opposed physical punishment of children, stating, "Harsh punishment of children is stupid."[43] Most
of his writing recommended tenderness, empathy, and diversion, although
occasionally his suggestions were more specific. At times he recommended
splashing a cup of water into the child's face or plunging the transgressor's
hands and arms into a bucket of water and letting them drip-dry.

His gentler alternatives to physical punishment did not always garner praise
from his readers—in fact, most disagreed. In response to "Obedience," a pam-
phlet written by Patri, one father weakly extolled it as "nice" but added, "I am a
firm believer in the wood-shed and I also believe that across your knees is very
nice quite often. . . . I believe that they should be taken across your knees and
their [underwear] removed and a good sound spanking applied, and that also
means boys, too."[44] About her misbehaving children, a woman from Missouri
wrote, "The less I whip the worse they get."[45]

The disagreements about the merit of hitting children was now seeping into
the private sphere of home life as family members began to disagree with each
other over this once cherished parenting practice. In 1938, a grandfather from
Ohio worried about his daughter who "whips" his grandson: "My daughter
has a very smart boy, two years old last December and I think they are very
unjust and cruel with him. . . . Common sense teaches anyone you can't beat
a good disposition in anything, even a dog or a horse."[46] A Missouri mother
with a 9-year-old daughter admitted to whipping her "only once in a great
while" but worried about her husband's harsher methods: "He whips without
reason when he does whip and I am always on nettles for fear of his making a
scene on the street or at the school building. I hesitate to tell him when she has
done wrong, for I hate to arouse his anger."[47]

In response to growing questions about parenting, one of the highest selling childcare books was published by Dr. Benjamin Spock in 1941, *Baby and
Child Care*, which counseled against the punitive child-raising practices of
earlier generations. Spock, a believer in firm and consistent parenting, did not
rule out spanking in early editions of his book. But he salted his manual with
concepts on the impact that parents have on their children's development, and
he introduced what at the time was a radical notion: Children are individual
little people, with their own unique needs, and the influence of parental upbringing is more important than previous generations considered. But this
shift is not without backlash or disagreement. While firmness still reigned as
important, the whip and rod were more often being replaced by a wooden
spoon, a belt, or the hand.

1950 to 1970

As mid-century arrived, a majority of parents still spanked their children lib-
erally. The idea of punishing out the willful or sinful parts of a child still lived
on in pockets of American society, while a more general support for spanking
found new ground. In response to the growth of alternatives to spanking
through "training," spanking advocates added a new twist and suggested that
children *wanted* to be spanked. Children hoped their parents would spank
them to ease their terrible feelings about their misdoings. One popular parenting book from 1952, *The Magic Years*, suggested that children kept an accounting of their misdeeds and wrongdoings and yearned for a spanking so
as to wipe the slate clean. It was the only way they could feel appeased by their
guilt.[48]

But uncertainty prevailed for many parents. In 1952, an article in a popular
magazine was titled, *Spank Him or Soothe Him?* Parents were unclear what to
do with a distraught baby or toddler.[49] But the answer was no longer a quick
swat and then sending them to bed. Instead of framing unruly children as the
problem, the focus began to shift to unskilled parents. Regarding a mother
who wanted to spank her 18-month-old daughter for breaking a precious
dish that had been left on a table, one psychologist said, "If anyone should be
spanked, it is the mother who did not have sufficient foresight to prevent the
conditions which produced such an occurrence."[50]

A 1964 book on parenting, *Children: The Challenge*, ushers in the concept that imposing parental will on children is futile—children will accept the punishment and continue to misbehave to assert their rights.[51]
Foreshadowing future problems, the author states that physical punishments
will rise in severity along with the children's will to do as they wish. While
suggesting mutual respect between parent and child, the authors assure
parents that if, even after learning new parenting methods, one finds themselves provoked to spank a child, parents should admit that it relieves their
own feelings of frustration.[52] Hitting a child is now coupled with the concept
of stress relief for the parent.

As the 1960s ended and the 1970s began, a movement for children's rights
was ushered in, following its predecessors of rights for people of color and
women. Not expecting similar rights to adults, the children's rights movement
focused on protecting children from abuse and neglect, ensuring dignity, and
optimizing opportunities for young people to develop their full potential.[53]
This children's rights movement quietly grew over time and lives on in society today.

1970 and Beyond

In the late 1960s public recognition of child abuse increased, and the long-held belief that all spanking is useful and warranted anytime a parent deems began to decrease. Guidance for parents on when to spank began to emerge, suggesting that some types of spanking are better than others. A 1972 parenting book states, "Simultaneous timing is important to establish the association. For example, suppose a toddler has just run out into the street. To teach him the danger associated with being in the street, the child's parent might give the child one sharp spank as he picks the child up out of the street. This spanking would teach the child to associate the middle of the street with danger, but a spanking after he is safely back on the curb is poor timing. The child should associate the street with danger; the curb, with safety."[54] Those in favor of spanking continued to tout its value, but they too began to suggest that there are limits on spanking. An intense and simultaneous tension regarding spanking begins. Two parenting books, both published in 1970 by respected child development professionals, reflect the deep divide. From *How to Parent*:

> Many parents also have the impression that modern psychology teaches that you should not spank children. Some psychologists and psychiatrists have actually stated this idea in print. However, as a psychologist, I believe it is impossible to raise children effectively—particularly aggressive, forceful boys—without spanking them. . . . [S]panking is a necessary and inevitable ingredient in raising psychologically healthy children.[55]

And from *A Parent's Guide to Child Discipline*:

> How often is it necessary to use physical punishment on children? The answer is *never*. But why do parents so often fall back on this "tried-and-true" method when "nothing else works"? The reason may be that momentarily the child is frightened into acquiescence, or at least he stops misbehaving. But most of the time physical punishment intensifies his determination to win in the end; though the parent feels relieved because he has gotten rid of his anger and frustration, the child feels only anger, humiliation and revenge.[56]

These new and conflicting evaluations of spanking made parents aware of a new phenomenon: spanking stigma. In response, spanking goes into hiding. The growing recognition that parents don't have to spank sends spanking into the quiet realms of family privacy. Child abuse awareness builds in the 1970s, and federal funds to prevent child abuse grow in the 1980s. The proclamation of Child Abuse Prevention Week in 1982 states, "[C]hild abuse and neglect cross all ethnic, social and economic lines. *Anyone* can be an abuser."[57] Effectively making any parent question their disciplinary practices.

The first inclination that spanking is not in the best interest of the parent began with the suggestion that it is physically hard to hold a child in place to spank the child. An author in a 1972 book states in *Changing Children's Behavior*, "Conventional punishments require too much work. For example, spanking requires a great deal of energy just to hold a squirming child in position. Few adults can keep spanking for more than fifteen or twenty seconds."[58]

In 1980 a European psychoanalyst, Alice Miller, called physical force in parenting a "poisonous pedagogy." Her book, *For Your Own Good*, questioned commonly trusted parenting practices that she named coercive: respect to parents simply because they are older, lack of respect for children simply because they are young, obedience makes a child strong, tenderness is harmful and will make a child weak, and parents are always right.[59] Miller surmised that "our status and degree of power determine whether our actions are judged to be good or bad."[60] Alice Miller built a case that beating children and spanking children is a hair splitting difference. "[W]e can protect ourselves from a poison only if it is labeled as such, not if it is mixed, as it were, with ice cream advertised as being, 'For Your Own Good.'" Miller's ideas were widely resisted. The acceptance of complete parental authority over children was so deeply ingrained that to question it seemed perverse. To make her ideas plausible, Miller used stories of tormented and dangerous adults to demonstrate the long-term implications of hidden cruelty in childrearing, connecting coercive parenting tactics to adult problems. Miller may be the first to suggest that parenting practices fulfill the immediate needs of the parent more than the child: the need to demand respect, to validate the parents' own upbringing by repeating it, and even fear of self-loathing qualities parents have repressed in themselves coming out in their child.[61]

In the 1980s parenting experts began to favor sadness and contrition for children's mistakes, and teaching kids how to make positive amends for their actions.[62] One popular parenting book, *Loving Your Child Is Not Enough*, related the story of a parent embarrassed and angry at her child's selfish actions. The mother spanked the child to teach a lesson. The author contrasted the story with a mother who responded calmly and took away an activity for punishment. Examples like this ushered forth parenting techniques that do not include hitting. One author provided a script for a parent to say after a spanking, seemingly knowing parents will have a hard time ending the time-honored technique of hitting a child for bad behavior. The script includes the parent apologizing for the spanking and quick forgiveness all around, with hugs and kisses to boot. And so, the movement away from spanking has a new foothold—parenting advice and examples with positive discipline or natural consequences—the two new parenting buzzwords of the time.

As the 1990s emerged, the majority of parenting books did not even mention spanking. The anomaly in this gaping hole was a 1994 parenting book, *Complete Book of Baby and Child Care*, which advised for disciplinary spanking, especially for "willful defiance."[63] The author suggests one to three swats on the buttocks or thighs, painful enough to cause tears and break down "defiance." Other books on childcare and parenting never mentioned spanking, even while the General Social Survey showed the continuing high rates of approval of spanking. Spanking, one of the most common methods of parental discipline ever invented, was rarely mentioned, as if it was a matter not to be touched.

A few parenting books advised against spanking. In 1991, Nancy Samalin wrote in her book, *Love and Anger: The Parental Dilemma*, "Parents always ask me what I think about spanking, and I tell them that if spanking worked, we'd only have to do it once. Basically, spanking is nothing more than a big person using force against a smaller person. It can do damage to your child, and in the long run, it doesn't work. You may be lucky and succeed in getting your child to obey you, or stop whining, or do what you want him to for a moment. But you've created hard feelings in the process, and you haven't set an example that you want your child to follow in the future."[64] In the 1992 edition of the very popular *Baby and Child Care* by Dr. Benjamin Spock, the long-regarded childcare expert suggested that parents try to avoid physical punishment. Even as he advised parents not to spank, he left the door open for the use of the technique; the rights of parents to choose, the sanctity of the privacy of the family, still reigned.

But not all parenting books published after 1990 ignore the topic. Spanking can still be found in the index of parenting books after this time, but it continued to drop until the mid-2000s, when parenting book indexes are nearly completely absent of spanking. In reviewing more than 100 parenting books (keep in mind there are thousands), I could not find any published beyond 1994 that advised spanking. The books didn't suggest a ban on spanking either. This common parenting experience was deftly and quietly being ignored, even while its occurrence in family homes continued at very high rates.

My lack of finding advice on spanking was reinforced by a sociologist's review of 10 widely used textbooks on parenting, which found that the majority did not have an entry in the index for spanking, or for physical punishment or any other synonym.[65] The top 10 parenting books previous to 1994 devoted, on average, only half a page to physical discipline.[66] It is as if experts didn't agree with it, certainly didn't want to advocate for it, but realized that to tell people they shouldn't do it might go too far. Maybe that's because even the experts themselves were spanking their kids and to tell others publicly they shouldn't spank would mean the disciplinary technique couldn't be used by them either. So we collectively avoided it, leaving it to families to determine in heated moments in the privacy of their home.

One of the advocates against spanking was SuperNanny Jo Frost's 2014 book, *Toddler Rules*. "You may not think spanking is wrong, but if you believe you have a right to spank your child hard and find a good excuse every time for why you do it, that's abuse."[67] Frost goes on to say that not only does fear not induce long-lasting behavior change, but that spanking does harm, even if the parent was spanked and turned out fine. She outright advocates, "Let's get the number of parents who spank their children to zero."

Mystery Misinterpreted

Over the centuries, perhaps the most influential source of support for physical punishment of children is the Old Testament in the Christian Bible.[68] The oft-quoted "Spare the rod, spoil the child" is not, in fact, a quote from the Bible but rather something of a summarization. The Book of Proverbs says, "The one who withholds the rod is one who hates his son" and, later, "Foolishness is bound up in the heart of a child; the rod of discipline will remove it far from him." There are about 10 other short biblical quotes that have been taken as proof that a Christian God supports spanking children.[69] Some Protestants reason that children are sinful by their very nature, and children who defy their parents may defy society and God Himself. Christians, especially Evangelical or fundamentalist Christians, are more likely than non-Christian parents to endorse and practice physical punishment.[70] They are supported by parenting books written by fundamentalist Christians encouraging spanking as an effective parenting tactic.[71] Some provided with zealous endorsement, stating that the rod should never be the last resort but the first choice, and with provocative book titles such as *God, The Rod and Your Child's Bod*.[72] Some claim the buttocks were created by God just for this advantage of a safe place to provide physical punishment, a highly sensitive area but not overly vulnerable to long-lasting injury.[73]

Dr. Stacey Patton in her book *Spare the Kids: Why Whupping Children Won't Save Black America*, states that the Black church continues to be a haven for sanctioning spankings. Black and Brown children have long suffered under the guise that a whupping is good for them.[74] In the name of God, and saving children from the evils of the contemporary world, are ideas fueled by ministers and pastors who suggest whuppings will keep a child close to the family and primed for learning and growth. This legitimizing spanking in the Black community as a God-given expectation forms a twisted knot with white supremacy. Patton interviews a Black Harvard Psychiatrist, Dr. Alvin Pouissant, who notes what the message really means: "They are saying that it's legitimate to beat Black children because they are lesser beings. And they're playing to white people by saying that their violence towards Blacks is okay because Blacks do it to themselves."[75]

Discipline and punishment, combined with religion, shape our attitudes towards power and authority for the rest of our lives as we carry them with us into the adult experiences of work and family life.[76] It shapes how we dole out our own authority and how we respond to others as parents, leaders, spouses, bosses, and friends. It shapes who we become as people of faith. The World Council of Churches, representing millions of Christian peoples worldwide, is directly opposed to corporal punishment of children. The Churches' Network for Non-Violence works to end all forms of physical punishment to children and directly challenges faith-based justifications for hitting children.[77] Biblical scholars have long expressed that the 10 verses identified as supporting spanking cannot be translated literally, nor can it be presumed that they are about an adult striking a child. These references, from the Old Testament portion of the Bible, may appear to support spanking but much less so when understood in the context in which they were written. Moreover, biblical suggestions of physical punishment are hardly limited to children, but we have chosen not to accept those in modern society. Intuitively, as a person raised in a Christian household, it seems a mischaracterization to say that God supports adults hitting children. Any act of hitting claimed to be done in the name of God is suspicious to those of us who understand a loving faith and how harm can be done under the guise of religion. Importantly, Jesus, who Christians believe to be the Son of God made manifest on Earth, never, in his recorded words, or his actions, ever suggested that inflicting pain on children, hitting them in any form for learning, was a method Jesus suggested or supported.[78]

Over the past 300 years there has been a slow decline in frequency, variety, and intensity of physical punishments inflicted on children. For any given family, in which raising children extends about 20 years, equivalent to one generation, the shift is imperceptibly slow. As government expanded its influence into the lives of children, such as outlawing child labor, making education mandatory, and intervening in abusive situations, the lives of children have improved.[79] As our knowledge of human development has grown, our view of children has changed, and our understanding of how parents influence the lives of their children have expanded.

3

Limits, Laws, and Little Mary Ellen

> Many people in our culture, if not all of us,
> speak the language of violence in one way or another.[1]
>
> —Gregory Moffatt

It was January 1874 when a woman who cleaned rooms in the Hell's Kitchen neighborhood of New York City noticed something disturbing, even for this troubled and impoverished neighborhood. The cleaning woman approached a church-based volunteer visitor, a precursor to the modern social worker, to express her concerns. The cleaning woman confided that there was a girl, Mary Ellen, being treated cruelly by her mother.[2] She was being beaten and had limited food and not enough clothing. The volunteer visitor felt compelled to act, despite no precedence for intervening in such a problem. The rights of parents to treat their child as they wished was so sacred that no one knew how to help Little Mary Ellen, despite the markers of physical abuse and malnourishment the cleaning woman had noted. The volunteer visitor attempted to enlist the help of others but found no partners who shared her urgency to intervene. She then consulted the founders of the American Society for the Prevention of Cruelty to Animals. Historically, the care of animals was placed before children in many parts of the world.[3] Animals met needs, such as labor and hunger, and children required additional resources and caretaking. The volunteer visitor persevered with her newly found partners, and they determined that the recently established animal rights laws could address the deplorable conditions of Little Mary Ellen. Using legal language they had developed to intervene in cruelty to animals, a legal claim was sought, and Mary Ellen was brought to court to testify in her own child protection case.

Little Mary Ellen, the first child abuse case in the United States, described a life of no stockings or shoes, a complete lack of affection, only a rug to sleep on, cuts and bruises from her mother's discipline, and fears of ever speaking to other people; the all-too-common isolation of abuse.[4] The court deemed her living conditions unsafe, and Little Mary Ellen was removed from her home,

Spanked. Christina L. Erickson, Oxford University Press. © Oxford University Press 2022.
DOI: 10.1093/oso/9780197518236.003.0003

as had abused and malnourished animals in the city of New York before her.[5] After this landmark case, the Society for the Prevention of Cruelty to Children was founded, based on the same conceptual ideas of preventing cruelty to animals. Other large cities followed suit within the decade.[6] A local police reporter made a prophetic statement, noting that this "marked the beginning of children's rights." The modern child welfare system was born in the United States. By the end of 1899 nearly every state had a Society for the Prevention of Cruelty to Children, and more than a dozen existed in other parts of the world.[7] Little Mary Ellen went on to be adopted by a loving family to and grow into old age with a family of her own. The story of her abusive mother is unknown, lost in the historical record, but likely included stigma and suffering.

Little Mary Ellen's story reveals the obvious abuse and coordinated effort required to first tear down the privacy walls of family life and intervene in the life of a child. The newly established societies began their philanthropic work with volunteer efforts over the next few decades, until professional, modern social work was developed. The acknowledgment of child abuse was given a leap forward when the 1935 Social Security Act provided funding to every state for child welfare services,[8] starting the beginning of professionalized, government-sponsored intervention for children's well-being. Nonetheless, it would be years before children who were physically maltreated would be given serious attention. It was not until the 1960s when a resurgence in public interest in child abuse emerged,[9] not because parent–child relationships had changed that much, but because public understanding was beginning to shift. What is identified as child abuse is culturally constructed in a time period. Child abuse is not so much about family brutality as it is about cultural acceptance in a time period of what is the appropriate discipline of children. Today's abuse is yesterday's punishment, and nowhere was this more clear than in 1962 when Dr. C. Henry Kempe identified the "battered child syndrome."[10]

The Battered Child Syndrome

The abuse of children was identified with Little Mary Ellen, but our understanding of some children's lives grew exponentially in the 1960s owing to the efforts of one pediatrician. Dr. C. Henry Kempe cared for children at Colorado General Hospital. After noticing children with unexplainable bruising and scarring during medical visits based on repeated "accidental" injuries, he became suspicious. He began documenting varying features on children with physical injuries, often repeated over a number of months or years. He took photographs of children's bodies, blocking out their faces for privacy, to show repeated scarring of a questionable nature. The photos showed scarring from abuse months previous along with current, fresh injuries. Many of these were on the buttocks of children, the space socially sanctioned for parents to hit. Some were in the shape of common household objects like a cord, belt, tree branch, or wooden spoon. Kempe's thorough documentation included the entirety of children's bodies with unabashed transparency. The pictures are difficult to view: burning on the buttocks and feet, fractured bones, tissue swelling on arms and legs, and scar tissue built up over time. Sadly, some of Kempe's photographs of child abuse were on children who had died at the hands of their parents. As difficult as this work was, he knew it could bring the issue of child abuse out of the shadows and into the national spotlight. Dr. Kempe's perspective on physical punishment became quite clear. In describing the physical disciplining of children, including spanking, he used the words "physical attack or child attack" to include any parental physical discipline to make the child behave.[11]

In 1962 Dr. Kempe and his colleague Brandt F. Steele published a manuscript in the *Journal of the American Medical Association* identifying a clinical manifestation they named the "battered child syndrome."[12] Dr. Kempe was deeply concerned that a national public health crisis was being veiled by long-standing notions of privacy of the family. Child maltreatment happens inside a family home, and access to these children was often only through an emergency medical visit. Parents rarely confessed to the abuse, often parlaying a story of falling off a bike, or out of bed. There are seldom witnesses. If there are, adult witnesses may corroborate with the abusers' story, for fear they will be in trouble too. Child witnesses may be afraid to tell or possibly never asked. The shame of child abuse shrouds the story, keeping all family members quiet.

Dr. Kempe's discovery spawned interest in uncovering the psychological variances between abusing and nonabusing parents. Psychologists began studying various factors to explain parents crossing the line from physical discipline to abuse. They could find no relationship between intelligence and abusing parents.[13] Those who abused their kids had the same range of intelligence scores as parents who didn't abuse their kids. When the abuse occurred, the parents believed that what they did was a normal disciplinary act to a child who was misbehaving. It seemed reasonable and appropriate. Moreover, they could not remember, nor could they describe accurately, the details of what happened when the injury occurred. It seemed like a normal spanking event, and how it shifted into abuse was unclear.[14]

Psychological researchers did make two important findings. Abusive parents did feel depressed, carried a sense of worthlessness, and expressed dependency needs of their own.[15] The abusive parents of infants often wanted to feel loved and cared for and expected to have their emotional needs met by the child, in ways that children cannot provide. The second finding was that parents who abuse their kids often have unrealistic expectations for their children.[16] They expected the child to do things that are developmentally impossible for their age, because of either brain development, motor control, or emotional maturity.

Sometimes, when a parent believes a child can perform a behavior, and the child does not, the parent interprets the child's behavior as defiant and unruly, thereby making the child worthy of receiving physical punishment. One stark example was a mother angry at her child for not feeding herself. Frustrated that her 6-month-old wouldn't even try to pick up a spoon, the mother perceived the infant as willful and lazy.[17] She physically punished her, and when the child didn't learn, the parent's actions accelerated and became abusive. The mother's lack of knowledge of child development was the real culprit for frustration, not the child. This happens at older ages, too. In 2016 a Texas man was upset that his 8-year-old son had missed a goal at a soccer game. He felt a spanking was in order and hit the child with a belt. The child estimated 10 to 20 hits, and the father estimated five to six. The punishment left welts and red marks, grounds for reporting the spanking as abuse. In response, the child protective system removed the boy from the family and brought him into supervised care.[18]

Other parental expectations that children have been spanked for that require an ability to meet developmental milestones include bladder control, following multistep directions, emotional control, making judgments in new surroundings, and the capacity to think about what the future might hold and respond to it. These developmental abilities cannot appear before biological readiness. The ages at which typical childhood skills begin have long periods of normal inception, but uninformed parents label the child as naughty, disobedient, or troubled. These at-risk parenting behaviors are often displayed by parents who were physically punished themselves, have a difficult relationship with their parents, describe their parents in negative terms, and may have low self-esteem or limited coping methods to deal with their own life beyond parenting.[19]

Out of these findings came interventions for child abuse, to educate parents to understand normal stages and ages of human development and to learn multiple discipline options.[20] Parents unaware of normal child development and lacking in parenting skills feel powerless. They can experience fear and anger in parenting their child, lose all sense of empathy, and interpret the child's behavior as disrespecting them. They often attribute inaccurate motives to their children, thinking the child wants to humiliate or manipulate the parent.[21] When it became clear that a common reason for parents to physically abuse their child was inappropriate expectations, Dr. Kempe clarified what he saw in his 1968 book *The Battered Child*:

> From direct observation of parents with children and the descriptions given by them of how they deal with their offspring, it is obvious that they expect and demand a great deal from their infants and children. Not only is the demand for performance great, but it is premature, clearly beyond the ability of the infant to comprehend what is wanted and to respond appropriately. Parents deal with the child as if he is much older than he really is. . . . We see two basic elements involved—a high expectation and demand by the parent for the infant's performance and a corresponding parental disregard of the infant's own needs, limited abilities, and helplessness.[22]

In 1966 California opened the first registry to take reports on suspected child abuse from the public. Within the first 5 months of opening, 1,679 families were reported for suspected child abuse. It was an unprecedented chance for new learning, and researchers gathered a sample of 421 families to study. They wanted to identify more clearly what was beginning to be understood as a "syndrome." How often does child abuse happen? Are there patterns? Are there experiences that precede the abuse? To deepen their findings, they completed smaller qualitative studies by interviewing families for a close look at family dynamics. Researchers concluded, "If all the people we studied were gathered together, they would not seem much different than a group picked by stopping the first several dozen people one would meet on a downtown street."[23] The families came from all economic backgrounds, though most were middle class. They lived in cities and rural areas; they were professionals and laborers; they represented a range of faiths; they were messy and neat; and while mostly White, they were also people of color. They were not necessarily mean or aggressive people. They were typical. "Soon we became aware that we were dealing only with the extreme of a much more widespread phenomenon."[24] They learned that many parents start with a typical spanking to change their child's behavior, but the initial impact is unsatisfactory, and the spanking is intensified. This is how the typical family, believing they have entered a normal disciplinary moment, find themselves abusing their child.

After publishing his findings, Dr. Kempe was ready to engage the public in understanding child abuse. Kempe's coining of the term "battered child syndrome," the most severe form of child abuse, led to a reawakening of experiences like Little Mary Ellen's. Kempe's work made a national impact. All 50 states passed laws requiring mandatory reporting. These laws required professionals, including teachers, social workers, nurses, ministers, and others, to report suspicions of child abuse or else find themselves to be vulnerable to prosecution for failure to protect a child. Kempe published more books and spearheaded the Kempe Center, still in operation today, to end the epidemic of child abuse through education and advocacy.

Kempe's efforts encouraged further social change. President Nixon signed into law the Child Abuse Prevention and Treatment Act in 1974 to "combat one of the oldest and most pernicious problems of society, a problem that has spread dramatically under the pressures of modern life. A million cases of child abuse are reported in the U.S. each year, probably only a third of the actual incidents, and at least 2,000 deaths a year are the result of child abuse."[25] While child abuse may be an old and pernicious problem, the "dramatic spread" was likely explained by growing public awareness, data collection, and the naming of the battered child syndrome.

A host of efforts to raise awareness of child abuse were initiated. A public service television commercial from the 1980s shows a young mom cooking in her kitchen, the phone ringing, and a wailing baby. As the food begins to boil over on the stovetop, her patience does too, and you see her approach her wailing baby with anger and frustration. The image freezes and a wise and domineering voice says, "Stop, count, breathe."[26] Many parents could relate, and the potentiality for abuse was universalized to the average parent. That mother in the kitchen with the screaming baby could be anyone. More than 100 women were interviewed at malls in Minnesota and Alabama about that commercial. A majority felt they could relate to the woman. Respondents felt the message was about being calm and in control, to pause and think, and to let parents' know you're not alone in your stress.[27] Given enough stressors, any parent could abuse a child.[28] Between 1976 and 1983, more $200 million worth of advertising was donated for public service announcements aiming to end child abuse,[29] including billboards on the side of highways, ads in magazines and newspapers, signs on buses and subways, and television and radio spots. The efforts worked. In 1971 less than 10% of adults in the United States felt that child abuse was a critical problem. By 1981 90% of people felt that child abuse was a "serious and widespread problem."[30]

Responsibility for the prevention of child abuse was set on a new site: the community. At the Third International Congress on Child Abuse and Neglect held in Amsterdam 1981, participants identified ways communities can prevent child abuse and neglect. They included flexible employment options for parents and outreach to school boards and health professionals, community clubs, and organizations to provide adequate child development education. It was a clear statement that parents alone cannot be blamed for harming their children and that social norms influence parenting practices, for harm or good.[31]

Home Is Where the Hitting Is

In 2011 a 3-year-old boy named Noah Fake was spanked by his mom and her boyfriend for wetting and soiling his pants. Noah's 26-year-old mother, Robin, and her 33-year-old boyfriend, Steven, were punishing the boy for his failure to use the bathroom on time. A misunderstood developmental skill is that bathroom management should be completed by age 3, and when children fail by this age, they are considered naughty. The abuse was led by Steven Neil without interventions from Noah's mom, Robin Grienke. The mom and her boyfriend "tossed him, spanked him, and punched him."[32] They put him in his room and proceeded to watch a movie and eat pizza.

It's possible that Robin and Steven rationalized the incident and explained the night's activity as a lesson learned. A good hard spanking, along with some additional discipline, and confinement to his room for the night would teach Noah a lesson about wetting his pants. But Noah needed medical attention, and the hours that passed until they brought him to the hospital were enough to end his life. Despite initially lying to authorities about what occurred, Robin was apologetic. Robin allowed a boyfriend to physically discipline her child; they both failed to empathize with the difficulty of potty training when you are only 3; and neither of them knew the difference between discipline and abuse. Noah had evidence of previous injuries, so physical discipline was likely normal in their family, but they had no prior experience with child protective services.

But when the physical discipline went too far, it was unclear to them where the line of abuse had begun. When does spanking become abusive—when adults misjudge their own strength and hit harder than expected, when they miss their intended target and hit a more vulnerable part of the body, when they unconsciously accelerate the hitting, when the child falls from the hit and is injured, or when the first spanking did not work and they attempt to reiterate their authority by continuing to hit the child for prolonged periods of time?

The point at which legal physical punishment shifts to child abuse is the "shade of gray" in spanking that has researchers struggling to find the holy grail. If we could identify what makes normal spanking turn into horrible child abuse, we can stop it before it happens. For a parent to determine what's reasonable during an important parenting moment is tricky. As one parent noted, "I mean—sometimes we felt like we were toward the point of getting like, abuse. But not really, because she never really got hurt."[33] Parents make difficult determinations during spankings. Using factors like age and size, parents quickly attempt to calculate the force of an effective but noninjurious strike when spanking. Other factors influence parents' spanking strike too, such as the seriousness of the child's misbehavior, the parent's anger, or how quickly the parent responds. Some parents spank to get the child's attention, and others aim to show the child who's in charge, to make the child pay for what they did, and to allow the parent to let off steam. Some spank because they don't know what else to do.[34] One parent who spanked too hard described the experience, "It starts out, I think, as honest discipline, and before you know it, you start feeling better as you hit and you keep going, and at some point it becomes nearly impossible to stop. After that happened to me, I began seeing the urge to spank as a warning—so I don't spank."[35] Many parents know about this risk of "hitting children harder than they intended," but many of them do it anyway.[36]

So how can a parent know they might be crossing the line into abuse? Thousands of substantiated physical child abuse cases were studied to identify when parents slip from discipline to abuse. But the findings were null. Nothing—not the age of the child, the gender of the parent, the parent or the child's abilities or functioning capacity, the economic stressors in their life—could predict when legal physical discipline switched to illegal child maltreatment.[37] It's not what many people think, like the caregivers intent to hurt the child, hitting body parts other than the buttocks, or just bad parenting.[38] It's not "those people." It is us. Child maltreatment occurs more often in families who use any physical discipline, like spanking. The more frequent the spanking, the higher the chance of maltreatment.[39] That makes sense: The more often you hit your child, the more often you have the opportunity to accidentally shift from discipline to abuse. Experiencing *a single spanking* increases a child's statistical odds to experience more severe violence by 3%, and if the parents use an object like a belt or wooden spoon, the odds increase by 9%.[40] A child who has been spanked as young as 1 year of age can have as much as a 33% higher chance of involvement in the child protection system by age 5 than a child who is not spanked that young.[41] As spanking continues, it becomes harder for parents to judge with clarity how much is enough and what is too much.

Dr. Kempe identified this way back in 1968; spanking children is part of a spectrum of hitting. "There seems to be an unbroken spectrum of parental action towards children ranging from the breaking of bones and fracturing of skulls through severe bruising to severe spanking and on to mild 'reminder pats' on the bottom. . . . Hence, we have felt that in dealing with the abused child we are not observing an isolated, unique phenomenon, but only the extreme form of what we would call a pattern or style of child-rearing quite prevalent in our culture."[42]

Child Abuse Laws

There are limits on what parents can do to children for punishment, and with good reason. They have extensive power over children because of their size and family position. Children are the only people who, in their everyday lives, can be struck by others, and the law does not regard it as an assault.[43] Violence toward children by the people who love and care for them is a significant problem. In the United States alone, about 3.5 million child abuse investigations are conducted each year.[44] Parents can legally use physical punishment at will in the United States, from birth until age 18. The moment the child reaches adulthood, it becomes assault.

Children are the only group of people in the United States for whom physical punishment is legally permitted. Parents are "entitled" to hit their children; it is considered unique from assault because of its context and purpose. Duty to the child and shaping of attitudes and behavior make hitting one's children acceptable because its aim is regarded as different from other hitting.[45] Other hitting may be to hurt, maim, or kill. The legality of physical punishment is based on the authority of a parent to teach and punish a child. Other positions of authority in society do not accept hitting as part of its purpose. Adults do not hit other adults for the purposes of correcting or teaching. Certainly not in the workplace. The legal support for spanking rests on the parent–child relationship, the age of the child, and the parent's purpose.[46]

Since the development of the national Child Abuse Prevention and Treatment Act in 1974, the view of what is maltreatment has broadened, and the definition of a spanking has narrowed. Mid-century, it would not have been uncommon for utensils, cords, or other implements to have been used in a spanking. When the modern child protection movement emerged in the 1970s, it planted seeds of the idea that children can be "at risk," even within their own homes,[47] and the identification of ways children can be abused has only expanded since then. While what is considered acceptable for a spanking has narrowed, meanings of spanking do not change steadily across time or geography, creating variety in social acceptance and child abuse determination.

State laws are based on the Federal Code, which defines child maltreatment as, "any recent act or failure to act on the part of a parent or caretaker which

results in death, serious physical or emotional harm, sexual abuse or exploitation."[48] The Federal Code is broad, allowing for a range of descriptions and
implementations in each state law. Each state and territory in the United States
has a unique legal definition of child abuse. Common legal language includes
"reasonable force," which allows for interpretation of the use of force to discipline children ensuring parental option to use hitting, not disallowing hitting.
Child abuse laws are adult-centered; they protect hitting. They are not written
from a child's perspective. A few states delineate specific parental behaviors
that are never appropriate, but these states are few in number. Reviewing
even a small sample of state laws shows the broad range of definitions and
identifiers for child abuse. Constant among them is the commitment of *intentional* physical injury that leaves a mark on a child.[49] The laws leave it to social
workers, police, medical professionals, criminal investigators, and sometimes
the courts to determine what is intentional and what isn't. What was reasonable in 1975 is not necessarily what is reasonable today. Factors that determine reasonableness for professionals include the amount of force, the extent
of the injury, the child's behavior that precipitated the punishment, the child's
mental state, and the child's age.[50] Even with these factors, determinations are
challenging.

There have been efforts to codify all spanking as a form of abuse. In 2007,
state representative Sally Lieber introduced a bill in California that outlawed
spanking before the age of 4, making it a misdemeanor. A backlash of anger
and hostility from parents across the state who feared intrusion into family
life ensued. The overwhelming demands placed on local police departments
if spanking were criminalized was a first line of complaint. Arnold
Schwarzenegger was governor at the time, and while he took no position on
the bill, he reportedly stated that he and his wife never spanked their four
children. Lieber's bill didn't make it through the legislature.[51] That same year,
a bill to ban spanking in the home was introduced in Massachusetts. Easily
defeated on grounds of privacy of the home and rights of parents, one local
radio host said, "What are you going to do? Are you going to have cameras in
houses? Are you going to have 5-year-olds testifying against their parents? It's
absurd."[52]

There is universal agreement that child abuse is unhealthy and dangerous.
Where spanking falls on the abuse continuum has been debated. We do know
that abused children live in families in which physical punishment is habitual
as part of their child-raising process.[53] We also know that spanking is the most
common and accepted form of physical punishment and raises the risk for
other forms of child maltreatment, such as psychological aggression and neglect.[54] What is the best measurement for determining physical child abuse?

One fundamental question is whether child maltreatment should be measured by the behavior of the parents or by the emotional and physical injuries sustained by the child.[55]

Protecting Children

The line between abuse and physical discipline is not as clear as one might think, and there are varied interpretations. Anyone can report child abuse, and some professionals are required to report. The most common reporters of child maltreatment are teachers and law enforcement at 40% of all reports, followed by social services at 11%, medical personnel at 9%, and the other 17% a mix of neighbors, friends, and relatives. Nationally, over 4 million referrals for 7.5 million children are made for potential child abuse each year.[56] Just more than half of these are found to be worthy of an investigation from social services. About 17% of those investigated each year find evidence of abuse or neglect, and the other 83% are determined not to be maltreatment.[57] Of these children who are investigated, gender is evenly split, but age is a different matter. The youngest are the most vulnerable. Children younger than 1 year have the highest rate of victimization. The most common type of child maltreatment is neglect, at more than 75% of the reports. This is followed by physical abuse and then other kinds of maltreatment. About 1,700 children die from abuse or neglect each year, and most of these children are less than 3 years old. The main perpetrators of child maltreatment, nearly 84%, are adults aged 18 to 44, with an equal mix of men and women.[58] The policy language in each state guides the investigative work, and the perceptions and culture of the local area shapes the assessments of the social workers who do the investigations. All of this allows for variations in how child abuse is handled. That can be okay. Often we want to be responsive to the communities in our local area.

Because state child maltreatment laws allow room for interpretation, professionals have developed aids to identify children who have suffered from abuse. Medical professionals have developed scores for patterns of bruising to try to differentiate normal from injurious bruising. Social workers have developed psychosocial assessment methods. Psychologists have developed interview techniques for children to encourage the telling of abuse. Abuse determinations require social, medical, and developmental histories to understand the child and parent.

When a child is reported with suspected child abuse, a local social worker must ascertain a myriad of variables that influence the life of that child. The younger the child, the greater the level of risk.[59] Injury to a small body by an adult is easier to accomplish, and younger children cannot defend themselves or even report the experience. Bruising and welts that appear on more vulnerable parts of the body, including the head, face, and genitals, are of higher concern.[60] The parents' abilities and limitations, stressors, family culture, and community; the chance of recurrence or escalation; the love and care provided by the parents; the network of family and friends for support; the parents' self-reflection and plan for future discipline; and observations of the parent–child interaction for evidence of love, fear, and affection all flow together to attempt to determine child safety and well-being. Sometimes the system works well; sometimes it doesn't. Overreporting of abuse is common out of fear for a child's safety. Fear of removing children from their home who shouldn't be is stressful. While across professions there is agreement on severe abuse, there are plenty of diverging thoughts about less severe incidents.[61] In later editions of Kempe's book, the authors state that assessing child abuse "remains unpredictable, a continuing source of uncertainty for parents, policy makers, lawyers, judges and society in general."[62]

Watching a sophisticated child protection social worker is an inspiring experience. Jan, a skilled and seasoned social worker, was my mentor in graduate school. In her early 50s, fit and small, she had a presence. She had worked in child protection for decades and avoided burnout and an angry personality by being the most settled person I have ever met. Her calm was intriguing. She moved quickly enough but never rushed. She treated everyone as if they were her equal, from the most struggling client in the poorest part of town to the "suits" who had power in government services. She never made anyone feel lesser than her, and she never acted like anyone was more worthy than her. It was effective.

That fall we visited the home of a teenage girl and her dad who were referred to child protection. The tension was palpable when we got to the home. But Jan was never intimidating, nor scared herself. When we explained why we were there, the dad was surprised but had no choice. We went into the kitchen and had a conversation. Jan asked questions, without stigma, that brought out the story. This dad was stressed, but as he talked the tension released. Jan empathized, but never pitied or patronized. He needed support. The longer they talked, the more aware and clear the dad became. Jan had brought calm and hope. The daughter wasn't in danger, they'd had conflict, more explosive than normal teenage–parent conflict, but he was doing the best he could as a single father.

It wasn't long and I followed Jan to a home with a similar story, teenage daughter and mom conflict this time. But after hanging out in the living room for a bit and visiting with the mom, Jan could sense the building tension, the nature and frequency of the conflict that had already happened, and the lack of empathy the mom had for the daughter. They needed a break from living together. The threat of more physical discipline was real, and Jan deemed the daughter's safety could be at risk. Jan had the daughter removed from the home and placed in foster care. Both of these families were White, working-class, single parents with teenage daughters, referred for potential abuse because of physical fighting and conflict. Jan walked a tightrope between safety and family unity. Across the nation, day after day, social workers make these tenuous and life-altering decisions.

Impacts on Parents

It can be scary for a parent to hit a child. Parents aren't typically going around hitting living things—knowing how much force is enough and what is too much can feel like hiking on a cliff through a fog. Parents can misjudge their strength, can miss their mark, and even be flat-out wrong. Very seldom can we take a hitting event and say that the person who did the hitting is 100% justified. Spanking is the only time we support and sanction the hitter and blame the victim. We even call it love. Maybe it is a kind of love, based on fear or shame rather than confidence. In many situations, parents spank their kids out of feelings of powerlessness. The child evokes in the parent a feeling of losing control, revealing their vulnerability, and the parent responds with a show of force. Powerlessness can lead to shame. Sometimes it's shame in the child and what the child has done, or sometimes it's shame at a parent's lack of influence with a child. Anger and shame may even be used as justifications for the actions taken by parents.[63]

For parents who were harshly parented or abused, spanking their child comes with its own baggage. Parents may fear repeating painful memories, and they viscerally understand the possibility of physical discipline that becomes too severe. One parent stated, "One time when she was about 4 years old, I had spanked her maybe a week before, and she had done something that made me really angry, and I wanted to spank her and she just like cowered away, and it made me feel like I was an abusive parent."[64] One thing shared by angry parents who feel like hitting but don't is the absolute knowledge that a spanking, initiated at the wrong moment, might turn into a beating. Some parents know this because it has happened to them.[65]

   Parent memories of shame or humiliation in their childhood spankings can deter parents from spanking,[66] or encourage it. A parent who was abused may find the familiarity of power and control either comforting or intimidating. Abusive family stories carry problems deeper than the physical bruises and scars they leave behind. Sometimes parents are trapped by their own histories into perpetuating parenting practices they don't approve of. Memories, long held and seemingly forgotten, can re-emerge when parents disciplines their child through physical punishment, diminishing the parents' ability to be responsive to their child's needs. What may start out as discipline can begin to feel like domestic violence. Imagine the parental fear when the spanking has gone too far, the fear of hurting their child, the potential report to child protective services, and the shame of social workers at their door to investigate the report.

In 1969 Jolly K. was a single mom with two children and challenging life circumstances. Struggling with trauma from her own childhood abuse, Jolly K. realized it affected her ability to parent. She physically abused her two children and was working to stop herself from abusing them more. Feeling her parenting was not improving despite her efforts, Jolly K. told her social worker that talking to other parents with similar issues might help. Her social worker, Leonard Lieber, set her up with another parent with similar experiences, and the idea of parents supporting parents was born.[67] The thrust of their idea was that parents can grow and learn from their mistakes and become better parents and people. They invited other parents Leonard knew to a meeting at Jolly K.'s kitchen table, and with a successful first gathering, the group decided to meet regularly. Members posted flyers around their community. They called the group "For Moms Who Lose Their Cool With Their Kids"— a meeting to share support and ideas. Their commitments to each other included stopping abusive behavior toward their kids, sharing phone numbers and being available to each other day or night, and welcoming others to join free of charge. "[B]y helping each other, they could find the strength to become the parents they wanted to be."[68] As the group grew, they moved into churches or any other free space they could find and called themselves Parents Anonymous (PA). The self-led groups had no fees or dues and promised no answers. Modeled much like recovery groups such as Alcoholics Anonymous (AA), the PA groups were facilitated by parents for parents. Anyone wanting support, information, or simply someone to talk to about challenges of parenting could receive help from PA. Like AA it was built on the idea of mutual aid; people in similar experiences sharing ideas were the best source of judgment-free help.

PA grew quickly because it appealed to a broad audience and underscored an important truth; parents are still growing too. "Through interactions with their peers, parents identify their options, examine their attitudes toward child rearing, and learn positive ways of relating to their children."[69] Joy in the "parental leadership" role was a main goal. Parents lead their families, and practicing how to do this was central to the PA mission. By 1980, PA had grown from Jolly K.'s kitchen table to 1,200 chapters serving at least 20,000 families. They shared phone numbers, which evolved into 24-hour helplines for parents to call with "explosive" feelings toward their children. As time passed and parenting interventions became more professionalized, some of the grassroots efforts of PA were lost. Eventually, PA grew into an international nonprofit organization with sophisticated training and services in collaboration with professional structures for child welfare, including the US Office of Juvenile Justice, which believed that confident and affectionate parents could reduce overall juvenile delinquency rates. They offered grants to PA, along with other formal organizations, and by 1980 the structure of PA had moved well beyond the parent-to-parent mutual aid that had nurtured participants from the beginning.

Jolly K.'s relationship with the organization she started had changed over the years. As PA professionalized with paid staff and educated advisors, the mutual aid that started the groups became just one part of a much larger organization. Her last role with PA was as a public spokesperson, but that contract was not renewed in 1981, ending Jolly K.'s role in the organization she had spent years developing. Jolly K. died of a self-inflicted gunshot wound at only 39 years old. A newspaper suggested that her sadness stemmed from her growing differences with the organization she founded.

Jolly K. 's honesty and openness, her willingness to share her vulnerability and face the stigma of parenting difficulties still has influence today. As one PA mom wrote, "The point I am trying to make is that Jolly K. and I had a serious problem and we needed help. Anger/rage issues are stigmatized, especially in women and more importantly in mothers, and was/is often swept under the rug, preventing those like us from getting the help and support we need to become the loving, successful parents we want to be. Through Jolly K.'s work to change important concepts, that help became possible."[70]

PA provides an interesting perspective; the focus is on the parent, rather than the child, in an empathic way. A dateless brochure from a California chapter, likely from the 1970s, asks questions as applicable today. "Are you a troubled or nervous parent who has no place to get help?" and "When you are ready to blow up is it you and the children who bear the brunt of it?" They offered the support of others who want a "family life more fulfilling . . . less explosive and tense . . . more loving." Jolly K.'s legacy removes the guilt and self-loathing that accompanies harsh parenting and the shame that keeps it shrouded in silence and allows it to continue. Jolly K. knew that to end child abuse and harsh parenting, children *and their parents* need to be heard, encouraged, and cared for.

The Nested Circles

We may think our private family life is not affected by the world outside our doors, but that defies the reality of the nested circles. Imagine a circle with you in it. Now, draw a slightly larger circle around that one. That circle includes your closest loved ones, often people you live with. Now draw an even larger circle around that circle. That's your next closest community, it might be your work or school, extended family, or closest friends. Draw a fourth larger circle and include your neighborhood, faith community, or groups you are part of and relatives you see less frequently. The circle beyond that one includes the state you live in and even your country.

What is in each layer of the nested circles varies for each of us, but we all have them. Each nested circle is linked and interacts with the others. Some interactions we see, and others we don't, but the ripple effect of each interaction reverberates through the nest. The people we live with have a big impact, and that's why they are in the circle closest to us. But the circles farther away matter too, and they influence how we think, feel, and behave.

While difficult parental pathologies are to blame for a small number of abusive families, the majority of families are trapped in situations where parental struggles and limitations are not countered by skills and knowledge in child development or support from professionals and their community. Healthy communities with close connections and support, healthy nested circles, have been shown to exhibit lower levels of all kinds of human violence, from child abuse to suicide.[71] We have risk and protective factors at the individual, family, neighborhood, and community layers of the nest, each in a complex interplay with each other.[72] What families need are more protective factors than risk factors that spread throughout the layers of their nests. If we have a violence-free life in one area, it buoys and is buoyed by other layers in the nest. The flip side is the same: Layers of violence in the nest affect the other layers.

Factors that potentially turn a spanking into child abuse can be in any of the nested layers. A family's stressors, including financial struggles, life events outside of the home, and the expectations and support of the community in which they live are influential. For the parents, it includes how they were raised, their expectations for their child, their nurturing capacity, stress levels, and influences from peers. For children, it includes their health and physical abilities, their temperament, how much care they need, and if they are more difficult than what the parent expected. Other forms of violence such as property destruction, domestic violence, and robbery are like a virus in the nest that spreads. Even witnessing physical violence is a risk factor for violence and makes one more likely to inflict harm on others. People can experience events that decrease their likelihood to participate in or be victimized by violence in the future too, such as loving relationships, community-building events, and positive adult role-modeling.[73]

Child abuse and other forms of family violence have been found to be more likely in communities characterized by chronic stress, concentrated poverty, fewer social supports, and low social cohesion.[74] If the rates of child maltreatment are higher, so are the rates of physical discipline because most incidents of child abuse start as efforts of discipline. Physical violence of any kind, to any family member, is a known stimulus of other violence.[75] Prevention means you avoid the risk. If nearly all child abuse starts with physical punishment, one of the best ways to end child abuse is to avoid the risk—by never participating in hitting a child.

One suggestion is to emphasize prevention of child maltreatment and promotion of family well-being by ending the acceptance of any form of hitting as a means of parenting.[76] In our current system, children in need of child protection are placed with foster parents who are prohibited from using any form of physical punishment.[77] Foster parents cannot spank the child they are fostering or their own children when a foster child is in the home. Even witnessing a spanking inside a foster home is thought to be traumatic to children. Perhaps, if given the same guidance and resources as a foster family, could the child not stay with their parents? Or, if hitting children were illegal, like hitting any other person, the child would still be at home because the hitting would have never happened.

4

Research and Revival

> "[Y]ou must realize that all of the leading psychologists and psychiatrists and educational authorities practically agree now that whipping a child is not the best way to make him obey or distinguish between right and wrong. . . ." But I did not state "my" point of view on spanking. I stated the Bible's point of view; and one word from the Bible is worth more to me than all of the words of the leading psychologists and psychiatrists.[1]
>
> —The Journal Mailbag, 1928

The crying lasted for hours. It was 6:00 p.m., and we were trying to have dinner with friends at their home. My 6-month-old daughter could not pull herself together. We changed her diaper, fed her, burped her, walked her, laid her down, put her in a swing, sat her up, nothing worked. Disappointed our plans were jilted, fatigued, and feeling crabby, we headed home early to deal with her crying bout. After more than 5 hours, she fell asleep. No explanation. No wonder technique found. Our pediatrician told us that crying jags, especially in the evenings, are common. "Just stay calm, try out your options, she will eventually stop."

Years later, perusing a parenting book I had bought titled *To Train Up a Child* (it had the sweetest cover of a grinning toddler holding a grown man's hand and a fishing pole), I read, "A seven-month-old boy, who failed to get his way, had stiffened, clenched his fists, bared his toothless gums, and called down damnation on the whole place."[2] My daughter had done that too, but the author's advice was very different from my pediatrician. Attributing motivations to this infant, the answer was to hit him with a switch, to assure the child knew he could not get his way. The book turned out to be a tour de force of when and how to use a whip and rod in spanking a child. If the child is manipulating you, and needlessly making demands, as the crying infant was doing, you teach the child to obey. There is no room for children's emotional needs or physical discomfort in this revivalist support for spanking. All

Spanked. Christina L. Erickson, Oxford University Press. © Oxford University Press 2022.
DOI: 10.1093/oso/9780197518236.003.0004

difficult behaviors of a child are rooted in explanations of badness, even in infancy. Obedience and surrendering to domination of the parents is a crucial element in loving parenting. Refusing to spank is a sign of weakness from parents who do not love their child enough. With a subtitled section, "God Spanks His Children," the authors state that those who refuse to use the rod on their child "are, by inference, condemning God."[3]

This zealous revival of spanking occurred simultaneously with growing research findings of negative outcomes. But through books like these, the revivalist notions achieved far better outreach than the research. The 1970s and onward saw an uptick in writing about spanking from both sides of the aisle. Much of it was driven by two well-educated men with deep similarities and deep ideological differences; Dr. Murray Straus and Dr. James Dobson. Both entered the spanking arena with fervor and zeal, albeit from vastly different perspectives and sources of information. Both men saw parenting as central to healthy child development. Straus, who had never been spanked was ardently against it,[4] and Dobson, who was spanked in abusive ways, was an ardent supporter of spanking.[5]

Dr. Murray Straus: Spanking as the Cradle of Violence

Dr. Murray Straus was professorial-looking in an absent-minded way— professional enough to wear a tie, too distracted to make sure it was on straight, and too involved in his research to care. Dr. Straus was a sociologist, professor, and researcher, with an openly identified Humanist faith tradition. I attended his presentation at a national conference where he spoke for more than an hour with densely packed PowerPoint slides in very small font. He emphasized years of research evidence on the negative effects of spanking to a mostly academic audience. He worked hard to jar the idea that hitting children can ever be normal. His family violence research began in the 1970s, and he is credited with identifying that violence is most often perpetrated by people we know and love, not strangers. He called the family the locus of love and support as well as the locus of violence.[6] The paradox fascinated him.

In the 1970s, about the time Straus began his research, and not long after Dr. Kempe's naming of the "battered child syndrome," the "battered woman syndrome" was identified.[7] It was social recognition that a spouse, usually a woman, could be hit, not feel safe to report it, and even think herself responsible for their spouse's actions. Battered woman syndrome pulled back the veil of private family life, shining a light on hitting a spouse as a form of violence. It sounds ridiculous today, but the realization that spousal hitting was criminal, and women are not responsible, was revolutionary. Straus worked to blur the lines between hitting a spouse and hitting a child in a time when family researchers and all of society considered the two acts completely separate. Straus saw no distinctions, recognized the wholeness of the family unit, and believed hitting anyone in the family was violence. He turned to diligent scientific methods to find proof. One of his early studies found that partners who are upset with a spouse are more likely to be physically violent if they were spanked as children. Followed by findings of increases in dating violence among spanked teens, increased rates of depression, physical abuse, crime, and even reduced economic income in adulthood were found for people spanked as children.[8] Straus diligently researched spanking, published his findings in respected journals, and presented at conferences like the one I attended.

Despite his efforts, Dr. Straus was concerned that his findings were met with apathy. Straus believed the hitting of children is so deeply normalized that his findings were largely ignored. High rates of family spanking had made it so commonplace that no one gave it much attention. Nearly everyone had been spanked or given a spanking, so it was not an interesting research phenomena.[9] Labeling the family the "cradle of violence"[10] and spanking the "virtuous violence",[11] Straus continued his message that spanking is the first and only sanctioned experience of human violence and begins right within our own families.

Despite his prolific record of research, 15 books, and hundreds of articles,[12] Straus sometimes felt shunned from the sociological community for his position on spanking. His main book, *Beating the Devil Out of Them*, was not a big seller.[13] Through his own description he was misunderstood by some of his academic colleagues. He described himself as a "a very socially concerned person, but . . . not a social person."[14] In the final years of his career, in his 80s, Straus published an autobiographical article describing the challenges from his own academic community about his work. He stated that his major research efforts were "bitterly criticized."[15] He believed that his stance that never, under any circumstances, should a child be spanked was found implausible. Straus noted a deep personal tension in his colleagues and other professionals—that even though they do not agree with spanking, they would never say it should not be an option for parents. His colleagues found Straus' ideas radical. He concluded that "the violence we so abhor and fear has part of its origins in the actions of loving parents who, by spanking children, unintentionally teach violence along with responsibility, honesty, cleanliness, and Godliness." In a dedication to Straus after his death, one of his colleagues wrote that he "was in an important way a moral visionary. He wanted to change the world. And he had a very inspired yet well considered hunch. It was that violence and abuse in the core institution of the family was the well-spring of much other human grief and adversity. . . ."[16] Straus died at the age of 89, his work ongoing.

Dr. James Dobson: Spanking as God's Gift to Parents

Dr. James Dobson claimed that his strict mother and the spankings with shoes and belts that he received from her are what saved him from youthful troubles. A child psychologist and a devout Evangelical Christian, his faith informed his clinical advice. He believed that spanking is a necessary act of loving parents. *Dare to Discipline*, first published in 1970, was a wild success, selling 3.5 million copies. Eschewing expert knowledge, Dobson stated, "The principles of good discipline cannot be ascertained by scientific inquiry. The subject is too complicated and there are too many variables involved."[17] His basis for the parenting advice he offered rested on common-sense parenting, Christian scripture, and ideas that "have been handed down for generation after generation and are just as valid for the twenty-first century as they were for our ancestors."[18]

Dobson balanced showing care for a child with absolute authority of the parent over the child. Dobson described children as willful, challenged, mocking, defiant, brazen, rejecting, and rebellious.[19] He felt listening to kids was dangerous because it allowed power to be given to the child to explain their point of view, reducing parental authority. Encouraging spanking, Dobson believed that the "pain associated with these events teaches him to avoid making the same mistakes again. God created this mechanism as a valuable vehicle for instruction."[20]

When a parent administers a reasonable spanking in response to willful disobedience, a similar nonverbal message is being given to the child. He must understand that there are not only dangers in the physical world to be avoided. He should also be wary of dangers in his social world, such as defiance, sassiness, selfishness, temper tantrums, behavior that puts his life in danger, that which hurts others, etc. The minor pain associated with this deliberate misbehavior tends to inhibit it, just as discomfort works to shape behavior in the physical world.[21]

Dobson's empathy for overwhelmed parents was limited. He compared a frazzled mom who popped out of her house at noon each day yelling at her children to a cuckoo clock.[22] "Weak old momma," and "poor, tired, old, dad"[23] are parental descriptors he used generously. He described children, even toddlers as "vicious and selfish and demanding and cunning and destructive."[24] Children acting in these ways were not time for discussion; he warned that only swift and full authority from a parent would produce positive results in the child.

Dobson was a powerful messenger, and his ideas had a huge platform with his international faith-based organization, Focus on the Family, and his radio show offered in 27 languages in 160 countries.[25] Couching spanking within a Christian doctrine, an existing moral framework that many people recognized, gave it an unarguable platform. It became what Malcolm Gladwell calls "sticky."[26] When spanking is cast as representation of religious faith, the behavior itself sticks. The association with religion holds the concept in high esteem and makes it hard to question. Spanking's simple technique, offered to frustrated parents, with so much love and hope at stake for their child, feels like a balm for their worry. An audience craving an easy answer for high-stakes outcomes, and the simplest of tactics based on faith, made for a message parents grabbed onto in droves.

With the publication of *The New Dare to Discipline* in 1992, Dobson clarified with emphasis that he does not believe in "parental harshness. Period!"[27] But he held strongly to his win–lose dichotomy of parenting, and a losing parent and a completely authoritative parent are the only options he sees. "Nothing brings a parent and child closer together than for the mother or father to win decisively after being defiantly challenged. This is particularly true if the child was 'asking for it.' "[28] Parents should welcome their child after a spanking with open and loving arms, and in this moment, when the child's will is broken, true heart-to-heart conversations can be had.

Followers of Dobson's clear advice queried him on what to do when spanking didn't work. Dobson doubled down on the usefulness of spanking, rather than suggesting other options. He reassured them that it was not the spanking that was not working but how it was administered. There are several reasons spankings fail, Dobson explains. First, the parent has not spanked frequently enough. If the child can sometimes get away with the behavior without receiving the spanking, the behavior will continue. Second, the parent spanks for offenses not serious enough, teaching the child that no matter what they do, a spanking will follow. The third is that they are not spanking hard enough, so the child feels no pain, and this is not a punishment. The final reason for spanking failure is that the child may simply be more strong-willed than the parent.[29]

Dobson does use facts and data in his 1992 version of *The New Dare to Discipline*; it is not all common sense and biblical scripture. In the first four chapters of his book, the ones on children and discipline, he has a total of four references, two of which are of his own work.[30] But most of the facts and data he shares are not about discipline or child development. He cites news articles on drug use, sex, AIDS, sexually transmitted diseases, contraceptive failures, crime, teen birth rates, and cruelty toward animals. He has 44 references about social problems, causing a rapid sense of fear and anxiety for parents. His language is fear based and inflammatory, and his answer to all these social ills is the clear and decisive discipline methods he offers. For struggling parents, it can sound like a reassuring answer to complex problems, even though the information on children and parenting is an echo chamber of his own ideas from two decades before.

Without Research or Revival

If there are moderates from this time period, they would be James Comer, Professor of Psychiatry at the Yale Child Study Center, and Alvin Poussaint, Professor of Psychiatry at the Harvard Medical School. In 1975 they published *Black Child Care* partly to help Black parents raise children in a racist society and to help White parents raise children with less prejudice. Covering the infant years through adolescence, they filled a void in parenting books that assumed a White-only readership. They identified outside pressures on families as stressors that leave less energy at home to be available to a child needing attention, resulting in quick parenting responses to stifle a child's demands.[31] Their second edition of the book in 1992, *Raising Black Children*, holds true to their first edition and expands on some new issues. Without shaming spankers, they ask parents, "If your child can achieve good control and behave well without spanking, why spank?"[32] Comer and Poussaint believe that in a loving home, spanking is unlikely to be harmful, but that its usefulness will soon end. They suggested that spanking children allows them to "pay their debt," the punishment is swift and tolerable, and their guilt for being naughty is relieved, but the learning is limited. Most important, Comer and Poussaint want parents to let children know they are disappointed with their actions through talking, and that they believe in them and know the child will learn to demonstrate responsible behavior. One problem with hitting is that by the time children grow up, parents won't have enough practice talking, and spanking will be far less effective. Dr. Comer and Dr. Poussaint lean toward assumptions that their readership has already spanked, without judgment. They advocate an ever calm response but conclude that simple childhood acts can get the better of parents sometimes, "and that's okay."[33] When you lose control and hit your child, apologize.

There is one change in the spanking sections in the two editions of Comer and Poussaint's books, reflecting the growing move away from spanking. In their 1975 version, they ended their section on spanking with, "Again, however, when there is love and trust between parents and children, spanking will not have a negative effect."[34] In 1992, they changed that line, in these otherwise exact sections on spanking: "Again, however, when there is love and trust between parents and children, spanking may not have a negative effect. But, in general, we do not recommend spanking."[35]

Research Findings in a Nutshell

When I first typed "spank" into a library search engine, hundreds of research articles were listed. I was intrigued by the breadth, depth, and quality of the research that had been conducted since the 1950s. As I read hundreds of articles, I saw that over many decades, researchers have expanded their statistical tools to manage the difficulties in analyzing spanking outcomes. The sample sizes have increased from a few dozen families to hundreds and even thousands. With ever more sophisticated methods of research (using larger sample sizes, matching study comparison groups, measuring data more than once, gathering data over longer periods, and using statistical means to control for intervening variables), researchers have identified causal links to these outcomes with significant certainty. The research findings included here are found in multiple studies, across a span of time, with statistically significant findings. The jury is clear: Spanking is a cause of several negative outcomes, and a "dose-response" matters. The more frequent and harsh the dose of hitting, the worse the outcomes.[36]

Childhood Behavior

It was 1957 when researchers first identified the link between children being hit at home and antisocial behavior and aggression toward others.[37] The repeated findings have continued since then. They've even been verified in studies of identical twins raised in different homes; the twin with

harsher parenting had more antisocial behavior.[38] Spanking causes what social scientists call, "externalizing behavior,"[39] research lingo for "kids being
naughty." This is measured through aggression-based behavioral problems,[40]
like being mean to others, breaking rules at school, not feeling remorse,
hitting or kicking others, and lying. All kids externalize their emotions to
some extent, usually anger, frustration, and disappointment. Any parent
knows this, and the triggers are wide and varied. Feeling hungry and tired are
common, but not being able to share, struggling to be quiet in an adult space,
being annoyed by other kid are other triggers, and the list goes on. Learning
to manage these emotions is arguably the most important task of childhood,
and the most important teaching role of parents. Spanking impairs the development of social-emotional skills in children, especially emotional regu-
lation and problem-solving skills.[41] Spanking at age 3, twice a week or more,
is predictive of higher levels of externalizing behavior at age 5.[42] Maternal
spanking is somewhat more predictive than paternal spanking of aggression,
likely because moms spend more time with kids and have more opportunity
to spank.[43] The more harsh and frequent the spanking, the higher the levels
of reported bad behavior, especially in the home,[44] where it can continue to
escalate.

As kids grow, we expect them to verbalize their needs, express patience,
and begin to think before acting. Kids who keep "externalizing" rather than
grow into communicating and problem-solving struggle to be successful
students, collaborate with others, follow directions, and respond kindly in
relationships. More troubling, if the parents' spankings are impulsive, the antisocial behavior portrayed by the child is more impulsive too.[45] The child's
externalizing increases the spankings, which continues to amplify the child's
externalizing behavior,[46] causing the spankings to grow harsher over time.[47]
A circular pattern has begun. The more the parents spank, the more they feel
the need to spank. If you combine that cycle with a diminishing sense of love
and joy in the parent–child relationship, it sets the family up for trouble. The
disciplinary practice parents used most consistently with boys with serious
externalizing behavior, like violence, were a lack of parental affection coupled
with spanking.[48] Long-term implications aren't much brighter. Oppositional
defiance disorder and conduct disorder are the labels placed on kids who
never mature out of their externalizing.[49] These diagnoses have outcomes that
land kids out of schools and family homes and into juvenile justice and mental
health systems. If you're dealing with a genetic predisposition to aggressive
behaviors, spanking is no salve. The aggression-producing effects of spanking
are enhanced if there are genetic risks to antisocial or aggressive behaviors,
especially for males.[50] And for some teenagers, externalizing transforms into

internalizing behaviors like anxiety, depression, and isolation[51]—all increased from childhood spankings.

Intimate Partner Violence

The first study connecting physical punishment as a child with domestic violence as an adult was conducted in 1974.[52] Although this was a small study of only 80 families, adults who had been spanked at least monthly had a higher rate of assault against their spouse. In 1977, a similar finding was found with 96 couples.[53] In 1990, studies expanded to include 2,143 couples, and the findings still held.[54] Research continued and discovered that physical punishment experienced as a teenager created an even higher chance of domestic violence in adulthood. By 1994, physical punishment was still a predictor of domestic violence even when controls for socioeconomic status, alcohol use, or age were applied.[55] Then it was discovered that partner violence starts before marriage, in the teen years. People physically punished as children are more likely to participate in dating violence.[56] Why does hitting evolve from childhood to romantic life? Normalizing hitting as part of family culture justifies the actions for adults. Spanking limits development of conflict resolution skills when young because there is so little talking and practicing of other problem-solving skills. Any physical hitting in childhood increases our chances for intimate partner violence as an adult, or violence in any other important relationship.[57] Finally, depression-based aggression can cause an adult to assault someone they love, like a spouse. Adults who were spanked as children tend to show higher levels of depression in adulthood.[58]

Health, Academic Performance, and Substance Use

Sometimes, through detailed methods, researchers discover downstream sequelae, meaning outcomes that occur later in life but can be traced back to an earlier incident. Researchers have to collect data for longer time periods and rule out other variables, but the results yield information on spanking impacts over the long term. Spanking's influence on mood, cognitive ability, and substance use has less research support compared with aggression, but the relationship is definitely present for this later life effect.

A 1975 study on the childhood precursors of drug abuse included 5,000 adults. As children, those who were spanked less than three times per week were less likely to become addicted to drugs and alcohol as adults.[59] But that's not the only disease affected by being hit. Years down the road, asthma, cardiac disease, and cancer are all elevated in adults who experienced physical punishment as a child and are worsened by higher doses of hitting.[60]

Physical punishment has been linked to decreased academic performance in childhood and lowered cognitive ability. High-frequency spanking in toddlerhood, more than twice a week, is associated with lower verbal capacity scores.[61] Physical punishment is related to declines in school engagement, and the harsher the physical punishment, the more likely the child is to seek isolation,[62] including from school. A big detriment is noted when spanking replaces the opportunity to talk about the behavioral mistakes and its impacts on others. It leaves a child learning that the misbehavior is all about them and their bad behavior, creating a sense that they are the problem and limiting the opportunities for change by practicing verbal skills and making reparations.

There is also a relationship between physical punishment and psychological distress and depression. Even very low levels of physical punishment, once or twice per year, contribute to feelings of distress for children.[63] Kids with more frequent hitting have greater distress levels. Unfortunately, high parental support couldn't buffer these feelings.[64] The findings follow children into adulthood, revealing a host of mental health impairments, including depression, suicide attempts, drug use, and heavy drinking.[65] Like the increased problems with aggression, the rates of depression, anxiety, and alcohol dependence grow with the frequency of hitting in childhood.[66]

Childhood maltreatment has been called the most preventable cause of psychopathology in adulthood, accounting for up to 45% of adult psychiatric disorder onset.[67] We've known since 2012 that harsh parenting, which does not qualify as abusive, is predictive of mental health impairments in adulthood such as mood and anxiety and personality disorders.[68] Through this research we know that all hitting, even what we have long considered benign and instructive spankings, are enough to account for a range of mental health disorders long past the spanking experience.[69] A person may imagine that the spankings given children are harmless, but no one wants to dally on this line. How much hitting is needed to cause these problems is unknown. What we know for sure is that accumulated spankings create a cascading set of multiple risks over time.

Explanations for Negative Outcomes

Before the 1960s, people's negative social behaviors were explained through theories on personality or drive forces that compelled humans to behave in certain ways.[70] Stemming from the "bad seed" idea, humans were believed to have an internal aggressive drive that was reduced when a person acted out aggressively. A kind of internal battery of aggressive energy needed to wear itself out. This led to early therapeutic ideas that by engaging in aggressive activities such as hitting a punching bag or a pillow, you can reduce the urge to be aggressive and can drain the anger and frustration out of yourself. This fueled the twin ideas that naughty children acted out of an internal drive and that spanking taught them a lesson and reduced parental frustration. But at least five studies from 1952 to 1969 showed that this idea was not supported in research.[71] Rather than draining the desire to aggress, aggressive behavior increased the more it was expressed. When people hit others, they charge their own and others' internal battery, they don't drain it. Social scientists determined that aggressive actions are self-generating; the more aggression a person experiences, either as perpetrator or victim, the more the person continues to participate in it.[72] Most aggressively parented children act aggressively, and much of the externalizing behavior that cause kids problems is learned behavior from their family home.[73]

Bobo Doll Experiment

In 1961, Albert Bandura was a 36-year-old psychologist at Stanford University. Bandura was interested in aggression and how humans learned to be aggressive. Bandura had a hunch that children learn to be violent by watching others—not from an internal and unchangeable drive. Bandura conducted an interesting experiment with children between the ages of 3 and 6[74] at the Stanford University Nursery School. Bandura divided the children into groups and placed a handful of children in various playrooms with an adult. There were multiple toys in each of the rooms, and one of them was a Bobo doll. Approximately 4 feet tall, Bobo was an inflatable doll with a weight on the bottom. After the doll falls down, it returns to the upright position. In one of the playrooms, the adult acted aggressively by punching, kicking, and throwing the Bobo doll. In the other room the adult ignored the Bobo doll and played with other toys. The majority of children who had observed the aggression toward the Bobo doll modeled the kicking, hitting, and throwing they had witnessed earlier, far higher than the group of children who had not observed that behavior. And, even months later, these children still acted aggressively toward the Bobo doll.[75] Naming his findings social learning theory, Bandura found that we repeat what we see others do, especially our first role models, our parents. Being hit and watching others get hit is a teaching mechanism; we learn from it. When children are spanked, they take that learned method of hitting into other relationships, such as with kids at the playground, romantic partners in adulthood, and eventually their own children in parenthood.

Most concerning of all was that children expanded on the original aggressiveness observed. Albert Bandura gives a synopsis of his findings while showing videos of the children acting aggressively toward Bobo. In a video available on YouTube, Bandura's voice-over states, "It was once widely believed that seeing others vent aggression would drain the viewer's aggressive drive. As you can see, exposure to aggressive modeling is hardly cathartic. Exposure to aggressive modeling increased attraction to guns, even though it was never modeled. Guns had less appeal to children who had no exposure to aggressive modeling. The children also picked up the new language that was more hostile."[76] Bandura observed that aggression confers power, especially within a hierarchy. Spanking and hitting provides a momentary feeling of power, seducing people into believing they have control in that situation.

Through the Bobo doll and other studies, Bandura showed that humans learn the behaviors of aggression. Bandura explained the four mechanisms of social learning theory in his 1973 book, *Aggression: A Social Learning Analysis*. He stated that attention is the first important mechanism. The person learning must want to pay attention to what the other is doing. People who garner the greatest attention are those with power, resources, and prestige. In a family unit, that is the parents. Second, the event is memorable, especially over a period of time. Spanking events fall into that category—many of us remember being spanked long into adulthood. Practicing the observed behavior helps the learning process. Children may hit their dolls, their siblings, others on the playground, and then a dating partner and finally their own children. Importantly, if the behavior is legally and socially sanctioned, like spanking, it is more likely to be continued. Bandura's social learning theory explains the intergenerational preservation of spanking, handed down like an old family recipe.

We can see how spanking has sustained itself over generations, but that doesn't tell us the whole story. There are other explanations, all of which hold some truth, for why spanking has such negative effects on the lives of children, and as this book postulates, on the lives of parents too. One central idea is that hitting causes loss of connection, severing love and trust between the parent and child. The child grows fearful of mistakes and no longer sees the parent as a source of support. This challenge to the parent–child attachment is reified each time a spanking occurs, further cleaving the bond of love and trust between parent and child. Another destructive mechanism of spanking is that people who are hit by loved ones often rationalize that they deserve the hitting. When the person hitting the child is a parent and the main source of love and authority in the child's life, the child justifies the hit by feeling deserving of it. In a twisted way, the parent aims for that justification; otherwise, the hitting would be considered morally wrong. When hitting reoccurs over time, those patterns of thinking kick in again. Feeling one deserves such treatment lowers self-esteem, making it difficult to be successful in other areas of life. Finally, families develop cycles of circular causality. Rather than stopping bad behavior, parents are supporting its growth. Parents and children find themselves unaware that they are encouraging the cycle of misbehavior and spanking. Like a treadmill, it is hard to get off. When hitting becomes a frequent form of discipline, a parent's sense of capacity diminishes, and if the child's behavior doesn't improve, the parent's frustration and shame grow. Bridged by parents' limitations in their disciplinary tactics and children's desire for attention, the cycle keeps repeating. Rather than change tactics, many parents buckle down and spank harder, leading to further misbehavior by the child and the potential for child abuse.

We need to grapple with these research outcomes: Being hit in childhood has effects across a person's life span. Feelings of frustration and anger from being hit by our parents can fuel unresolved anger that comes out in adult relationships. Anger toward a spouse may include hitting, or if we feel we have limited recourse with a spouse, it may get taken out on our children. The verbal lashing we were forced to accept at work may ignite our sense of disrespect, with the smallest infraction from our child firing up a backlash. In the book *The Body Keeps the Score*, Bessel Van Der Kolk describes how distorted bodily messages can make it difficult to detect harmful situations from those that are safe and nourishing. The message that hitting children is loving is a profound example of that distortion. Van Der Kolk says that when we can't adequately self-determine what is beneficial or harmful to us, we often repeat unhealthy behaviors to assuage difficult feelings.[77]

How happy or smart would kids be without being spanked? We can never know. For kids who are spanked very young, it is even harder to see the potential losses in development. While the degree of negative effect is hard to quantify for a specific child, there are almost always negative effects of spanking—simply because a child is being hit by someone who loves them.[78] Calculations have shown that ending child abuse would significantly reduce depression, alcoholism, suicide, substance use, and domestic violence.[79] Hitting children hurts in more ways than one.

Does Spanking Work?

Not really, or at least not in the way parents hope for, and certainly not better than other options. Part of the appeal of spanking, the reason it has sustained over multiple generations, is that it appears to work in the short term. The child stops the negative behavior at that moment. It feels like a successful parenting event. But the devil is in the details. Behavior change does occur in young children for a short time after a spanking.[80] Human behavior, however, rarely responds consistently. So while the spanking worked in one time and place, and the child stopped that behavior, it won't work every time in every situation, often diluting the impact over time. This requires a ratcheting up of the spanking so that it will work again. Sort of like fast food, you get a quick, easy meal and feel full, but the negative effects play out farther down the road. Those negative effects layer on each other, like pounds on our waistline. The most detrimental outcomes of spanking are found in older kids and in longer time frames away from the spanking experience, and because of this, the effects are harder to see.[81]

The years between ages 2 and 6 can be the most challenging for children to comply with adults' requests, and it is this age range that physical punishment research is most documented. One belief parents hold to justify spanking is that children's compliance with parental requests at younger ages often reduces more severe discipline later.[82] A child who quickly stops the offending behavior does allow more time for the teaching of new behaviors.[83] Hitting is often used to quickly stop a child's behavior, but it isn't the only option. Kneeling down to look them in the eye or removing a child from the situation can be just as effective. Even by age seven, withdrawal of privileges or additional chores works better than a spanking.[84]

Here's a good example of what can fool parents into thinking that spanking works. Forty moms kept track of how often their children had disruptive behaviors such as sibling fighting. Spanking or a conversation with reasoning stopped all fighting for 9 hours on average. If the reasoning is combined with a punishment such as a timeout, privilege removal, spanking, or a hand slap, it more than doubled the time until the next bad behavior, to more than 19 hours.[85] Thus, a conversation with reason along with a timeout or removal of privileges works equally well at stopping sibling fighting, completely eliminating the need for spanking. More important, there are no negative outcomes from a reasoned conversation or a timeout; there are none for removal of a privilege either. Also important is the parents' own growth and development. There is no shame from hitting—only conflict resolution skills, good feelings of role-modeling, and no risk of harm to the child and the ensuing worry of professional interventions.

In all fairness, researchers supporting spanking have advocated for a clean delineation between mild and infrequent forms of spanking and harsh and frequent spankings, suggesting that the negative outcomes are from severe spankings only.[86] They suggest that spanking may not be the culprit; harsh parenting is. It is true that a mild spanking applied with a conversation in an otherwise loving and close family will likely not be as detrimental as a harsh spanking in a family with fractured relationships. If we follow this debate, the spanking delineations become quite granular. What is too much spanking? What hitting is harsh? There is a spanking threshold.[87] When corporal punishment becomes harsh, or the child feels a sense of injustice, its negative effects are stronger. If parental rejection is part of the equation, the outcomes are even more detrimental. The question then is, do parents and children agree on what is harsh? Or too much? Most compelling of all, there are no long-term, positive outcomes related to spanking. There is not an increase in desirable child behavior over time, nor is there an improved internalized understanding of positive social behavior. There is not a single positive long-term benefit to children or their parents that can be attributed to spanking.[88]

What Is Meaningful?

The research assistants sat quietly in family homes. Blending into the background, they turned on their audio recorders, observed, made notes, and tallied. They counted every word spoken from parent to child and child to parent. They noted tones of conversations and how family members responded to each other. They closely documented family dynamics. Over a 6-year period they quietly watched and observed inside the homes of 42 families. The lead researchers, Hart and Risley, verified the data through long hours of audiotape analysis and review of transcriptions. The data gathered were full and rich. Such depth and specificity in qualitative data is rare and illuminating. The researchers, coming from the fields of child development and psychology, were deeply intrigued by young children and the experiences that shape their behavior and language development. After all, behavior is communication, especially for young children.

They discovered that the number of parents' words and their tone shape their children's communication in profound ways. Parents spoke the same number of words to their 8-month-old as they did to their 3-year-old. Not surprisingly, the children began to speak like the parents. If what they heard was "shut up" or "move," that is what the children said when they were old enough to speak. If their parents gave a longer explanation, children followed that pattern too.[89] When parents talked more, they often encouraged the kids to explain themselves and ask more questions. Kids learned to talk as much as their parents. As soon as the number of words they used matched their parents, they did not add more, and they continued to talk the same amount as they learned in their home. It wasn't just the number of words though, it was also the style and the ways of interacting. Hart and Risley found that the words parents used are full of emotion. Rarely do parents speak in polite, monotone conversation to kids. They almost always instruct, command, cajole, disapprove, or encourage. These constant interactions, filled with emotion, set the tone of the relationship and create a kind of "reservoir" of feelings to draw on between parent and child. Hart and Risley reported, "By the time the children were three years old, trends in the amount of talk, vocabulary growth, and style of interaction were well established."[90]

Observing family dynamics, they found that the words and tone chosen influenced future behavior. Positive or negative tones from parents promoted similar communication patterns from children. "When we listened to the children, we seemed to hear their parents speaking; when we watched the children play at parenting their dolls, we seemed to see the futures of their own children." At three years of age the mimicking of tone was striking. Parents who gave 80% of their feedback to their children in a positive tone had children who spoke positively to their family members 70% of the time. When 80% of parental feedback was with a negative tone, 80% of the children's tone to family members were negative.

All the families in the Hart and Risley study were free from serious problems. None were involved in child protection. All but one of the families used spanking, and many of the children were given timeouts for misbehaving. All the children were developmentally on target for their age and were preschool-ready. Each family took care of their kids, nurtured them with food and clothing, and showed love. Across all these families, the parenting activities were remarkably similar. The difference was that some families conversed with their children beyond what was necessary to provide care.

The families that spoke the most, on average, recognized their kids' positive behaviors 32 times per hour, and gave a verbal reprimand, telling them what not to do, about five times per hour. The families who spoke the least recognized their kids' positive behaviors on average five times per hour, with 11 verbal reprimands in that hour. The families with a negative tone spoke less overall too, so the ratio of negative reprimands to positive comments was far higher than in families who spoke more. They didn't talk to their kids a lot, but they did talk to them when they had to, such as when they were doing something dangerous or naughty. This lends itself to a lot of, "Don't do that," "Stop!" When children in the study misbehaved, parents gave kids explicit verbal disapproval of their behavior. Most spankings are accompanied by such a verbal reprimand,[91] and these often include verbally disparaging remarks. Spanking is a form of communication without words. It doesn't require explanation or allow for the child to talk. In fact, that could be perceived as sassiness or talking back, encouraging more spankings. When the spanking is the communication, there is no room to practice difficult conversations, for the parent or the child. When parents spank they become an enforcer, not a family leader. It robs them of the chance to practice conflict resolution and dialogue, articulate a solution, show hope and love, demonstrate leadership, and offer the opportunity for growth and change.

Parents can dress and feed their children, teach them skills like potty training, hold them accountable for inappropriate behavior, and still not fully engage them as if they are interesting and valued individuals. When children receive parental interest nearly always as corrective or critical, it shapes their world. One of the most powerful tools for shaping and changing the behavior of children is positive reinforcement. It's simple at its heart. Parents put energy and attention into positive behaviors that their child is displaying. What is rewarded is repeated. Child development experts encourage parents to respond to children when they are behaving well, not just when they are behaving badly. This encourages the "positive opposite of the unwanted behavior."[92]

Spanking also doesn't encourage joint problem identification and problem-solving—so much of what we hope our kids learn to do as adults. This kind of joint problem-solving involves talking to people with more authority than you, articulating your experience, and describing how you are learning and growing. As a college professor, I find that the students who do well are skilled at talking: first, about their assignments and grades, then about ideas and their own dreams, and finally about what else human society needs to know or learn to improve lives. The students who avoid me, don't feel comfortable talking to people with power, struggle the most.

Parents can provide the first practice zone for meaningful conversations with others, including those with more power and authority. As kids age, we need to be able to discuss problems with them and attempt to solve them through verbally mutual benefits and maintain an emotional relationship. Parent–child relationships that can do this with warmth promote social competence.[93] The only true alternative to action, including hitting, is words.[94] Words help us understand, reflect, assess, evaluate, emote, and gain a new perspective. Words are meaningful.

Things We Haven't Researched

Research on spanking centralizes the experience of the child. Parents are made nearly invisible in a discourse that is primarily about their actions. Like men being erased from the conversation about violence toward women, parents have been erased from the discourse on spanking. Jackson Katz in his Ted Talk on *Violence Against Women: It's a Men's Issue*, clarifies why. "This is one of the ways that dominant systems maintain and reproduce themselves, which is to say the dominant group is rarely challenged to even think about its dominance."[95] Katz continues, noting that one of the key examples of power is the lack of necessity for introspection. The way we think about spanking conspires to keep us focused on the child and what they did wrong and not on the parent's emotional state, hitting behavior, or alternatives that may be better. Spanking research that focuses only on children renders impacts on the active person, the parent, moot.

I could not find research that studied the impact on the parent of spanking one's children. The lack of interest in parental impacts stems from dual beliefs. One is that children are developing and can still be shaped by the spanking experience. The second belief is that adults are developmentally complete and not affected by the discipline methods they choose to use with their children. These two beliefs manifest in research that focuses on the child and ignores the adult. Humans most often become parents in their 20s. Research tells us our human brains don't even reach maturity until age 25,[96] an age at which many people have already become parents. The majority of our life comes *after* we start our families. After we have already started spanking our children. People are just launching roles as citizens, professionals in a chosen career, and budding leaders. Brené Brown says in her book, *Daring Greatly*, "It's a terrible myth to believe that once we have children, our journey ends and theirs begins."[97]

If researchers had studied the effects of spanking on parents over the past 50 years we might have a different perspective. I changed the titles on a sample of research articles on spanking to be parent-centric. I removed the words "child" and "school" and replaced them with "parent" and "work." Researchers would have had a different story to share had they studied *Corporal Punishment and Parental Behavior and Cognitive Outcomes; Strengthening Causal Estimates Between Spanking and Parents Externalizing Behavior Problems; Dimensions of Physical Punishments and Their Association With Parents' Cognitive Performance and Work Adjustment;* and *Slapping and Spanking by Parents and Its Association With Lifetime Prevalence of Psychiatric*

Disorders. My own experience is that how I discipline my children significantly shapes me. I can't find a study to back up my claim, but it intuitively feels right.

Early childhood is a special time. Children effectively parented will often attain positive results in their adulthood, including less violence, higher achievement in work and academic endeavors, reductions in health disparities, and most important, happiness.[98] What is missing is recognizing young childhood as a special time in the lives of parents too. Parenting isn't a static activity: Parents grow, change, and develop much like their kids. Having had one bad parental moment is certainly not a reflection of all parenting activities, and the fleeting moments of feeling like you're doing the right thing can be just that, fleeting. These parental changes are understudied by researchers, and their impact on the developing personhood of the parent is only beginning to be understood.

How does spanking affect parents? What is the impact of an adult hitting a small child's body? This is what I set out to learn, and I can't definitively answer it. Parents who stop spanking have been shown to quit because they had a personal change of philosophy about hitting, their spouse disagrees with them, it resurrects negative memories of their own upbringing, or they see that the spankings negatively impact their child.[99] No research has studied whether parents found spanking to be negative for themselves. And so I propose that spanking is bad for parents.

Research on spanking is valid, but it is bound. We can't research mystery, it's hard to describe love, and a scientific understanding of the human spirit is yet to be determined. Science can't reveal everything and has even been described as a specialized way of being wrong.[100] Sometimes, we simply ask the wrong questions. Conceptualizing hitting our children as useful for learning is just the way society has described it so far. So fill in the blanks with your philosophy of life, your understanding of moral obligations, and soul searching on what is right for the young people you care about. *And, what is right for you.*

PART II

5

School Paddling

The Only Legal Place Beyond the Home

With Alexa Anderson

> Children are the only citizens regularly subjected to physical punishment.[1]
>
> **—Andero & Stewart**

The shiny birch paddle in the woman's hand was about 4 inches wide, 10 inches long, and one-quarter inch thick. Two women, in business casual clothes, professional and well kept, look experienced and assured. They are addressing a 5-year-old boy. The small boy standing in front of them is wearing khaki shorts, a camouflage jacket, and tennis shoes. He has a tousled mop of sandy hair. His head is lowered, he is whimpering, and soft, muffled pleading drifts up toward the women. They are in a well-appointed office, with wingback chairs, a plush rug laid over the industrial carpet, and floor-to-ceiling bookcases lined with books that wrap the walls. The women lean over to hold the boy, and in a kind and gentle tone, explain that the boy needs only one paddling, unless he squirms, for failing to follow directions and spitting. The boy cries and wriggles, begging not to be hit. The child's mother, Shana Perez, is recording the event on her cell phone without their knowledge. The boy is given one whack on his clothed buttocks, screams, and cries, and the punishment is over. Shana claimed that her son had two options: take the paddling or be suspended. The child had already missed 18 days of school. In an interview later, Shana tearfully stated that her son hates school now. This is Jasper County, Georgia, United States. The year is 2016.[2] Repeat much of this scenario in Florida in 2021. A mother secretly videotaped an elementary school principal paddling her 6-year-old daughter for scratching a computer screen. The mother reported the incident to the police, but the Attorney General found no crime was committed. The principal stated the mother had consented to the

Spanked. Christina L. Erickson, Oxford University Press. © Oxford University Press 2022.
DOI: 10.1093/oso/9780197518236.003.0005

paddling, even though the mother denies she understood.[3] Paddling is an accepted and utilized form of school discipline in the United States.

History of School Corporal Punishment

Corporal punishment in schools, synonymous with physical punishment, has a long history, much of it chronicled in European boarding schools dating back to medieval times. Physical punishment then could be banishment to a small room or withholding meals, but generally speaking, it meant being hit, usually with a whip or a tree branch, sometimes referred to as a switch or a birch. In the 1700s, early philosophies on student learning believed that obedience was so important that education was nothing more than learning to obey those in authority. Beatings and whippings were sometimes described in early educational manuals and books without much fanfare. There was an absolute acceptance in the right of teachers or principals to hit a student at the their discretion. Whippings for speaking out of turn, or not speaking in English, were common and expected in colonial days.[4] Whipping and paddling children were believed to be a useful intervention for all kinds of youthful problems, as well as a motivational tool for learning. As time passed, the whip, switch, and birch were replaced by a wooden paddle. Throughout the 1800s, paddling by teachers was commonly expected, with no impunity for the teacher and school, no need for consultation with parents, no documentation of the event, and no option for another type of discipline.

1867—New Jersey bans corporal punishment in public schools.

Some of the earliest research efforts published in the leading *Journal of Education* revealed that students believed paddling a worthy discipline. In 1895, a schoolmaster in Sioux City, Iowa, conducted a typical research project of the time, one I saw repeated in library archives. He told a story to his 5- to 7-year-old students of a naughty boy who needed punishment: "A boy named Charlie threw down his pencil during math class and said in an angry voice, 'It's no use. I can't do this number work!' After being encouraged by the teacher, Charlie still refused to try." The schoolmaster then asked his students, "What should the punishment be for Charlie?" In all these early studies, the whip and paddle are chosen by the students themselves, supposedly affirming student support for the disciplinary practice. In Charlie's case, 666 students out of 1,021 said Charlie should be whipped, licked, or spanked.[5]

Published in journals read across the country by early professionals, the expectation of whipping and paddling in school by teachers and administrators was commonplace.

Innovation played a part in school paddling too. Spanking multiple children in a day can be quite tiring for the spanker. A school in Kansas developed a solution for this fatigue: a special chair to assist with the discipline. The Electric Spanking Chair was unveiled on February 14, 1898, at the Girls Industrial School of Kansas. It was built high enough from the ground to allow for paddles to be operated by electric wires. Straps were used to hold the students' wrists to the arm of the chair, assuring the girls would stay in place. Misbehaving girls were strapped in the chair, the attendant simply pressed a button, and the chair did the rest, relieving the spanker of the physical labor of spanking. Schools in other states, such as Colorado, considered ordering their own chair.[6] School paddling was wholeheartedly accepted as part of a sound educational environment.

The first major study on school corporal punishment, completed in 1902, was titled *Corporal Punishment in Twenty-Five American Cities*. Claiming that the whip was used less and less each year in schools, the study identified who is allowed to give physical punishment, how it is reported, and how parents are informed.[7] Those three elements remain salient today in school paddling. The 1902 report described the variety of rules and techniques utilized in school corporal punishment at the time. For example, several states required that no students could be hit on the head, and San Francisco allowed only straps or rattan in their paddling, with a complete exemption for paddling girls. In Providence, Rhode Island, written consent from a parent had to be obtained before a paddling could ensue. In Milwaukee, it was forbidden to "shock innocent pupils by the sight of the chastisement," mandating that the punishment be done in private.[8]

A panel of school professionals publicly debated the merits of spanking in 1929. In what must have seemed progressive for the time, the Louisiana State Superintendent stated that he believed that school paddling was outmoded 100 years previous. His emphatic request was to help prevent students from misbehaving to stop school paddling. Another superintendent stated it was degrading to the teacher and he would never allow it, and another claimed its lack of originality and usefulness made it unwarranted.[9]

From the 1930s through the 1960s the publications regarding spanking in schools faded. School paddling continued, quietly supported and common. Sometimes, in an air of paddling pride, children were made to sign the paddle they were struck with.[10]

1971—Massachusetts bans corporal punishment in public schools.

In 1972, the National Education Association (NEA) appointed a group named the Task Force on Corporal Punishment in Schools. Members represented various regions, urban and rural communities, students, and teachers. After a year of discernment, the Task Force on Corporal Punishment came to the following conclusions: Teachers and other school personnel abhor physical violence no matter what the form. No teacher wants to inflict pain on a young student. Teachers use corporal punishment only when the ways of dealing with disruption are poor and the school staff is very frustrated. The Task Force recommended that all educational systems move immediately to phase out corporal punishment, within 1 year, beginning in the 1972–73 school year. Despite their deemed authority, the recommendations of the Task Force went unheeded and were never acted on.[11] The acceptance and normalization of corporal punishment in schools was simply too strong a tide to turn.

1973—Hawaii bans corporal punishment in public schools.
1975—Maine bans corporal punishment in public schools.

In 1975, the American Psychological Association, in a public statement, opposed the use of corporal punishment in schools. The statement gained little to no traction. The majority of psychologists at the time believed spanking was a useful parenting tool, used it in their own families, and felt it was effective for school personnel too.[12] The acceptance of spanking was so culturally ingrained that even though in professional circles psychologists opposed hitting children, that did not translate into institutional changes, or even personal ones. The potential for child abuse and the negative outcomes of paddling were not enough to influence school professionals to take a stand.[13]

Despite their limited influence, efforts continued, and a year later, in 1976, a national meeting of the American Psychological Association Task Force on Children's Rights and Child Abuse hosted a public debate on school paddling with influential education professionals, medical doctors, and psychologists. In an effort to bridge the contentious divide, the moderator began, "All of the individuals involved in the symposium debate are honorable men and women. That they disagree so vehemently with each other attests to the importance of both sides attached to the practice of spanking children in the public schools."[14] Those speaking on behalf of paddling reiterated their abhorrence of child abuse. Lansing Reinholz, Superintendent of the Burlington Vermont Public Schools, defended his argument:

Do you wish to receive corporal punishment, or do you wish to be thrown out of school? Those are the last two alternatives we've got. Which one do you want? I can tell you that in the 13 years that I've been a school administrator and a school teacher I can recall and document at least 200 instances of corporal punishment. That's not all whacking. That's not all using paddles. But, if you shake a student, if you grab a student, if you wash a student's mouth out with soap, that's corporal punishment. If a teacher grabs a student by the ear to make him/her do something, that's corporal punishment. We're not talking about things limited to spanking. In all of those instances where I've paddled children as a high school principal, I've never once failed to offer the child the alternative of being suspended from school, permanently. We're not talking about a 3-day suspension or a 10-day suspension. And never once has that independent thinking child chosen to be suspended from school because he/she wants an education. He/she wants to be someplace where people care what the hell happens to him/her. And, in most of those instances, they choose the corporal punishment because they know that we do care; and in many of those instances they come from homes where the parents don't care.[15]

Reinholz qualified his support of paddling by noting that corporal punishment decisions should never be made based on race, gender, or economic factors. Statements like, "that's the only language they understand" or the child is "beaten at home" should not support the use of corporal punishment in schools. Reinholz finalized his argument with, "A pampered child from an affluent home would be more likely a person to benefit from a 'slap on the ass.'"[16]

Debaters supporting paddling in schools connected the discipline of paddling to the prevention of larger social problems, like drug use, crime, and even lack of motivation. There were no data to prove these lay theories, but the anecdotal evidence and the long-held traditions of paddling clung to such reasoning. Significant support for paddling rested with the belief that the only other option was school suspension. Suspended students would be vulnerable to the lures of the streets, and a paddling would allow them to stay in the safer school environment. Hitting was the last resort.[17]

Dr. Kenneth Newbold, a superintendent from North Carolina, spoke frankly about his support for corporal punishment. Wanting to assure the audience that North Carolina was keeping up with modern psychology, he named several alternatives to spanking they used and stated, "We are not a backward state."[18] He had used corporal punishment as a teacher and as a principal and found it effective, especially in grades kindergarten through sixth. Newbold argued in the debate:

I am the first to admit that corporal punishment can fail with some pupils and that it could be psychologically harmful to some students. However, in my experience, I have never seen evidence of any lasting psychological damage as a result of the use of corporal punishment. If it is reasonable and if the teacher does not administer it in anger or in front of other pupils, it can be a very effective tool with most students. . . . In the last seven years, the national Gallup poll has ranked discipline as the number one concern of parents in America. . . . [S]chools are a victim of an overall lack of respect for rules and authority. The lack of discipline is identified with some of educations foremost problems: crime, parental neglect, apathy towards school activities, idleness and lower academic standards . . . .We have excellent discipline in the school systems of North Carolina, and I attribute a large part of this outstanding record and good discipline to our state law that allows us to use corporal punishment when all other disciplinary measures fail.

Later in the debate, to bring a corporal punishment scenario to life, Dr. Gertrude Williams raised a paddle over Lansing Reinholz, and accused him of cussing, which he had done in the debate. She grabbed him by the arm, "Now then, Mr. Reinholz, you have cussed in this classroom. You have used the words *ass, damn,* and *hell,* and I'm going to give you a choice, boy! You have a choice of quitting your job or getting hit across your ass with this corporal punishment stick, and it's not going to be done by me, babe, because I'm angry at you! It's going to be done by Dr. Welsh."

Reinholz replies, "I'll take the stick!"

Dr. Williams' effort to demonstrate the foolishness of paddling may have landed flat or have been the moment of reckoning. Either way, she continued, focusing on racism and "reverse sexism" in school paddling, identifying what was yet to be shown in the data, that boys and children of color are paddled more frequently than girls and White children. Aiming to point out the absurdities of hitting, she proclaimed with incredulity to the audience, "[A] child striking a teacher creates disorder, yet a teacher striking a child creates order?"[19]

1977—Rhode Island and the District of Columbia ban corporal punishment in public schools.

Not Cruel or Unusual

On April 19, 1977, the US Supreme Court, in a 5–4 vote, ruled that school corporal punishment does not violate constitutional rights, specifically the

Eighth Amendment that prohibits cruel and unusual punishment. The Eighth Amendment prohibits imposing painful physical punishments in criminal justice systems and was specifically designed for those who were jailed or imprisoned. School systems, and the students in them, are not bound nor protected by the Eighth Amendment. Despite the long history of corporal punishment, broad public knowledge about the occurrence of school paddling was minimal in 1977. Little data was kept, and it was not possible to show the courts how expansive or problematic school corporal punishment was.[20] The case that brought the issue forward to the Supreme Court was not convincing enough in 1977, yet it feels shocking today. The 1977 Supreme Court ruling that upholds the right of schools to use corporal punishment on children was based on the case of James Ingraham vs. Willie Wright.

It was October of 1970 in Florida, USA. James Ingraham was a 14 year old boy, an eighth grader at Drew Junior High school. The morning started in the school auditorium, maybe for an all school event or announcements. At the end of the event students were requested to return to their classes. James and other students were requested to leave the stage of the school auditorium, and James was slow to exit. Because he was slow to leave the auditorium, he was sent to the principal's office of Mr. Willie Wright. Once there, James protested that he should not be punished because he was following the teacher's orders. Wright considered James defiant and determined he needed a paddling. Wright called in assistants, two male school administrators, to help with the paddling. Both men held James by his arms and legs face down across a table. Wright, using a traditional wooden paddle, hit James across the buttocks at least 20 times. James returned home to his family and required medical attention for his injuries. He needed a week of bed rest, laxatives, and pain relievers, and missed a week of school. James was not the only story of corporal punishment that came from Drew Junior High. Others were similar. Students were paddled for small infractions, while denials of culpability led to harsher punishment. Even brass knuckles were used on schoolchildren.[21] The Court noted that Drew Junior High used excessive force and caused damage that was degrading to students.[22] Despite these reports, medical professional testimony, and testament from students at the school, the Supreme Court upheld a school's right to use corporal punishment, citing, "Faced with this evidence of what is considered appropriate by the American people, we would be loath to suggest at this time corporal punishment is unacceptable to contemporary society." The vote of 5–4 was close, and the judges against corporal punishment spoke out against it with vehemence. They argued the lack of fit with modern teaching, punishments more severe than the offense, potential for injury, lack of justification for such severe methods of punishment, and children's lack of rights for protection.[23]

The Judges who voted to uphold corporal punishment in schools felt that to outlaw corporal punishment "bucks a settled tradition" of school paddling. Since only a handful of states had banned corporal punishment in schools by 1977, there appeared no movement to end the tradition. The Court did require new safeguards. Physical punishment should not be used as a first penalty, it should only be used with a prior warning, and another school staff ought to be present for the paddling.

When coercive practices have for so long been ingrained in our schools, homes, and other social institutions, we have normalized them as common practice,[24] and we don't know them as bizarre until someone using them in these common settings takes them too far. The Supreme Court reaffirmed this decision in 2011 when an eighth-grade student in Mississippi, who was paddled by his school administrator, fainted and fell face first on the floor, breaking his jaw and five teeth.[25] The student and parent filed a lawsuit but made no progress. The 1977 ruling of *Ingraham v. Wright* sealed the conclusion that schoolchildren cannot be protected under the Eighth Amendment of the Constitution, addressing cruel and unusual punishment. Prisoners and jail mates are free from corporal punishment, but children are not. Paddling an adult prisoner is degrading enough to be offensive and outlawed, but the court once again, did not agree that paddling a child in school was cruel.

One conundrum is that school personnel are allowed to leave bruises and injuries but parents are not. Why? Because of the immunity clause. Thirty-one percent of states that allow corporal punishment have legal protections written into the law stating that those designated to administer corporal punishment will be immune from civil and criminal liability if acting within district policy guidelines. As in Alabama, where legal language states, "So long as teachers follow approved policy in the exercise of their responsibility to maintain discipline in their classroom, such teacher shall be immune from civil or criminal liability." It's very difficult to prove unreasonable use of force with an immunity clause.

1983—New Hampshire bans corporal punishment in public schools.
1985—New York and Vermont ban corporal punishment in public schools.

In the early 1980s a school psychologist, Nadine Block, was working in Ohio. She was stunned when she discovered the principal using a paddle with children in the school where she worked part-time. Unwilling to let it continue, she began an organized movement to end school paddling in Ohio. Much of her work involved galvanizing and even comforting parents whose children were paddled. Parents were unsure if they had any recourse. Her discoveries and her strategies are chronicled in her book, *Breaking the Paddle: Ending School Corporal Punishment.* Nadine Block went on to found the Center for Effective Discipline[26]. Her work spanned many years of advocacy, coalition building, and awareness of the harms of corporal punishment, much of it through stories and photographs documenting family's experiences. Parents reached out to the organization when they found they had no recourse with the school or the school board, which shielded teachers and administrators from any negative recourse.[27] Often the first place these advocacy groups referred families to were medical providers to document the injuries sustained from the paddling. Psychological help was often next, and many families desired apologies to their children.[28]

It was in 1985 that the National Parent Teacher Association wrote and adopted a resolution opposing corporal punishment in any school, anywhere.[29] At their national convention they passed a resolution on corporal punishment in schools, stating that "the National PTA establish a position opposing corporal punishment in accordance with the Health and Welfare Policies of the National PTA; and be it further that The National PTA and its state PTAs urge units and councils to work with local school districts to develop disciplinary procedures which will result in positive behavior of students and to utilize techniques which are not based on physical abuse."[30]

1986—California bans corporal punishment in public schools.
1988—Wisconsin and Nebraska ban corporal punishment in public schools.
1989—Virginia, Oregon, Minnesota, Michigan, Alaska, Connecticut, North Dakota, and Iowa ban corporal punishment in public schools.

In 1990, Dr. Irwin Hyman, a school psychologist and the director of the National Center for the Study of School Corporal Punishment, described the outcomes of being physically punished at school in his book *Reading, Writing and the Hickory Stick.* Hyman identified the lingering stress and trauma of school corporal punishment on children and named its impact on students "educationally induced post traumatic stress disorder" (EIPTSD). Similar to PTSD from war, Hyman noted that children who had experienced traumatic disciplinary tactics have symptoms such as sleep disturbances, concentration problems, and personality changes, and they re-experience the trauma of the discipline in and outside of their school day.[31]

1990—South Dakota bans corporal punishment in public schools.
1991—Montana bans corporal punishment in public schools.
1992—Utah bans corporal punishment in public schools.
1993—Illinois, Nevada, and Washington ban corporal punishment in
*   public schools.*

Modern educational philosophers have taken us a long way from expectations of total obedience. Touting educational experiences such as critical thinking, expressing opinions, identifying evidence, and evaluating research findings, modern education has evolved from the early years that encouraged obedience, memorization, and rudimentary skills in reading, writing, and arithmetic. Education researchers and advocates have made the case that the potential negative educational impacts of physical discipline far outweigh any rule compliance followed in a single school day. For example, 90% of the college-bound students from states that allow school paddling had American College Test (ACT) scores below the national average.[32] Additionally, because of the overrepresentation of students of color in paddling, physical discipline should be considered partly responsible for the academic achievement gap between groups of students, especially students of color and White students.[33] Over the decades, the goals of education have changed, and so have the methods of instruction. But vestiges of historical eccentricities remain, including school paddling.

Some schools reinforce paddling in the privacy of the home; for example, they can require/request parents to spank their child for school infractions. Six-year-old Chandler was required to be disciplined by his school for excessive talking and acting out in class. Schaumburg Christian School in Illinois had a policy that parents spank their child for school infractions. But Chandler's mom felt she wasn't being true to herself as a parent and felt taking away privileges was a better option than spanking Chandler. The school's written disciplinary guidelines included parent-administered physical punishment as a requirement of the school. When Chandler's mom refused to spank the child, he was suspended.[34]

2003—Delaware bans corporal punishment in public schools.
2005—Pennsylvania bans corporal punishment in public schools.
2009—Ohio bans corporal punishment in public schools.
2011—New Mexico bans corporal punishment in public schools.

Contemporary School Paddling in the United States

"The best way to get the country in shape again is with our Make Kids Great Again wood carved paddle!" An online store sold the wooden paddles, hand-carved with an American flag and the words, "Make Kids Great Again," along the length of the paddle.[35] Varnished with a polyurethane coating, it shines, and the hand-carved and darkened distress marks give the ominous sense that it would hurt if put to use. The individual crafter selling the items is willing to add a personalized script too.

Nineteen states continue to allow physical punishment in public schools, many using wooden paddles like these. In 2018, estimates are that 100,000 to 200,000 young people were paddled or hit each year in public schools in the United States.[36] Corporal punishment is allowed in private schools, always has been, and they have their own long history of physical punishment. Two states ban corporal punishment in private schools: New Jersey and Iowa. There are no data collection systems for private schools, so these figures are unknown.

Jared Abrams grew up to spank his kids, and he found it didn't work. He realized he was spanking because that's what happened to him, not because he wanted to spank. He recalls entering the fifth grade and knowing the teacher paddled anyone who misbehaved. "The fear of going into that class stayed with me my entire life." *The Board of Education*[37] is a short documentary film by Jared Abrams describing paddling's contemporary manifestation in schools. Abrams' film shows school personnel striking students, in front of others, with belts and wooden paddles. He interviews coaches, school administrators, and teachers, claiming that having even one paddled child sent a message to other kids to stop their bad behavior. But there is fallout to the child as well as the teachers. Abrams' documentary provides the numbers of students paddled in each of the states, along with teachers and psychologists discussing the negative impacts on school culture. Abrams shows pictures of the bruises from school paddling; they are shocking. One teacher admits that it may not even have been the paddled kid that frustrated or angered the teacher, but the teacher takes it out on a singular child, and worst of all, kids know this.

> *2019—Mississippi bans corporal punishment for students with disabilities in public schools.*

The first collection of data on rates of school corporal punishment, from a sample of national schools, occurred in the 1975–76 school year by the Office of Civil Rights (OCR), a division of the US Department of Education.[38] As a result of data collection differences across school districts and a lack of uniformity in what is collected, it has been difficult to draw out comparisons over the years. Likely, not all cases of paddling are reported to the school administration, the school board, or the district office. Sometimes, school districts fail to collect the data.[39]

In 2005–06, when additional efforts were made to gather data on school corporal punishment, it was learned that hundreds of thousands of children were disciplined using physical means, one of the most common being paddling with a wooden board. In that year alone, from just a sample portion of the students, 38,827 Alabama students and more than 59,429 Texas students were physically punished in school. Overall, more than 260,000 students were physically disciplined in school.[40]

The OCR is the government-funded body that compiles data on corporal punishment in schools. Unfortunately, the data are unlikely to reflect the full portrayal of corporal punishment. The OCR data are drawn from self-reports from school districts. As noted in a five-page document titled "Data Notes" describing corrections made to the data in the 2013–14 school year, incidents may be underreported by schools because of reporting and measurement errors, such as "definitional difficulties, the inability of respondents to provide accurate data, differences in the interpretation of questions, errors made in collection (e.g., in recording or coding the data), and errors made in estimating values for missing data."[41] The data gathering includes only the number of students punished, not the number of punishments. Students physically punished multiple times would only be counted once.[42] The data notes for the 2013–14 discipline report state that "users should carefully consider the caveats for analyzing the state and national estimates included in this document." Moreover, data on school corporal punishment was not included in reports to Congress or the public, limiting transparency of physical punishment in schools.[43] In that 2013–14 academic year, it is estimated that 110,000 public-school students received corporal punishment in the United States.[44]

Research on outcomes for children who are paddled in school, which has been studied worldwide, is only recently understood, but the findings are similar to those for physical punishment in the home. Things that matter in school, like reading, writing, and mathematics, suffer when kids are paddled, and it affects their testing skills and their verbal skills.[45] The "externalizing problems" continue too, like defiance, aggressiveness, and verbal opposition. Studies show that school corporal punishment increases the odds of violent behavior and aggressive conduct.[46]

2022—States that allow or protect corporal punishment in public schools are Alabama, Arizona, Arkansas, Colorado, Florida, Georgia, Idaho, Indiana, Kentucky, Louisiana, Mississippi, Missouri, North Carolina, Oklahoma, South Carolina, Texas, Tennessee, and Wyoming.

Legal Language

The federal government leaves educational policy largely to state decision-making bodies and local government entities. Public schools operate in a complex system of local discretion, supported by state mandates and authorized through federal laws that require states to offer schooling, and each level of government provides some funding for meeting specified requirements. This localized system creates a wide variety in the quality and practices of public schools. The intention of local school control is that community input will help shape school board policy that best reflects the will of the community.

The legality for corporal punishment in US educational settings resides in individual state legislation. Thirty-one states have banned corporal punishment in their public school systems. Two states have no specific language on the matter, and the other 17 states provide varying specificity of legal language on how corporal punishment may be administered. In each of these states the length, content, and detail of the legislation varies. Some state laws grant schools the ability to use corporal punishment in just 24 words, others use 1,589 to describe the lawful act, including who can deliver the corporal punishment, if their must be witnesses, and sometimes the exemption of liability for school personnel. Ironically, this exemption allows school personnel to punish in ways that would be abusive if done by a parent. Teachers and principals in these states are mandated reporters of parental child abuse, but no one is mandated to report corporal punishment by teachers and principals.

One might expect definitive guidelines on how to safely paddle youth within a school; however, the legislation for many states is short-handed and sometimes vague, using terms such as "reasonable force." Emphasis on the immunity of the teacher, school, and school boards from civil and criminal liability stands out. When coupled with the lack of a definition of what corporal punishment is (only four states define what corporal punishment includes), there is enormous room for interpretation. Even today "corporal punishment" is an umbrella term that encompasses a spectrum of physical punishment to the human body, from a slap on the hand to being paddled with a wooden board. In Tennessee, the legal language allowing corporal punishment is broad: "Any teacher or school principal may use corporal punishment in a reasonable manner against any pupil for good cause in order to maintain discipline and order within the public schools." Seventy-four percent of these states identify who in the school system is allowed to give corporal punishment, about 10% of states require that another staff member be present, and about 37% require communication to parents in some form. In some states and districts, parents may have to give written or verbal consent every year, or verbal permission before the child is paddled for an infraction. Sometimes a child can only be paddled once per semester, and in some places, it is only allowed in elementary schools and is banned in middle or high schools.[47]

In the 19 states that allow school corporal punishment, individual school boards and school districts can affirm or disavow paddling. Local decisions can also include who can administer, for what reasons, and how delivered. Like spanking inside the family home, shame and stigma can shroud paddling in schools. Parents fear talking about it, even if they disagree with the school. It could embarrass their child or other family members. Parents may find themselves, or their child, ostracized by families who think paddling is a necessity for school discipline. Families who silently disagree with school paddling may fear getting involved.[48] Like the unquestioned assumption that a spanking parent is always right, a paddling school principal may not be questioned either. When spanking is valued in the family home, community support will often fall in line with the school paddling, even if the paddling was overused or unjust.

Inequality

Paula Flow, in a 2008 interview on National Public Radio (NPR), shared the following story: "I've been teaching since 1980 in New York City, that's where I started, and it wasn't until 2006. . . . When I had gone to Georgia, that was my first time witnessing children being corporally punished. The teacher asked him had he done his homework and he said no, and she popped him in his head with the palm of her hand and I said, can I take him to the library? I was just getting to know him. I tested him, he couldn't even read all of the letters of the alphabet. But he was a special ed. fifth grader. And I was in shock."[49]

School corporal punishment is not doled out to children equally. First, it depends on where you live. If you live in Montana, it's illegal to hit children in schools, and it's not allowed in New Mexico, but if you live in Florida or Georgia or North Carolina, it's an option for you. And if you live in Mississippi,

Alabama, Arkansas, or Texas, it's more likely than anyplace else you live in the United States.[50] Boys, overall, have received far higher doses of corporal punishment in schools since tracking of these data began in 1976.[51] Black boys receive corporal punishment about twice as often as White boys and Black girls and three times as much White girls.[52] Tragically, like Paula Flow's comment, schools may assess a child's behavior incorrectly. Evidence suggests that students are physically punished for symptoms related to their disabilities, especially autism, obsessive-compulsive disorder, and Tourette syndrome, all disabilities with which the children do not have complete control over their physical, mental, and emotional abilities.[53]

Like most people, administrators' own upbringing influences their paddling beliefs, but also fear of reprisal, their job experiences, and expectations of parents influence their choices about corporal punishment. Many administrators who use paddling still see punishment, even with its contradictions and compromises, as "in-service" to education and school culture, not as a conflict.[54] Paddling is often justified by school personnel because suspension is thought to be the only alternative considered for school infractions and is considered harmful to the child's learning. Paddling may appear to decrease violence and keep a child in school in the short term. But it can also increase insubordination and decrease academic aspiration,[55] which will lead to decreased attendance in the long run. Neither suspension nor corporal punishment is needed for school infractions, and there are a lot of alternatives, many of them focusing on positive disciplinary techniques.

Inside a school, corporal punishment often occurs swiftly, with only decision makers who are inside the school building, and without outside oversight, making schools the only organizations that allow hitting other people to be supported and silenced inside the walls of that institution. Reporting of these incidents can be spotty. Often these local entities are the monitoring and data-keeping sources as well. This arrangement can create a lack of recourse for families. There is no objective body to turn to. When the same institution grants permission and monitors, there is wide room for misuse. Importantly, public reporting requirements do not include severity or level of harshness to the student. One researcher studied stories on physical punishment in schools and found that the harshness of the punishment was not related to the severity of the misbehavior. Students were just as likely to need medical attention for punishments due to minor infractions as they were for serious school violations.[56] Fortunately, paddling rates in schools have fallen. After reaching a recorded height in the 1980s, rates have fallen from more than 5% of all children to closer to 1%.[57]

In *The Body Keeps the Score*, Bessel van der Kolk states, "It is standard practice in many schools to punish children for tantrums, spacing out, or aggressive outbursts—all of which are often symptoms of traumatic stress. When that happens, the school, instead of offering a safe haven, becomes yet another traumatic trigger. Angry confrontations and punishment can at best temporarily halt unacceptable behaviors, but since the identifying alarm system and stress hormone are not laid to rest, they are certain to erupt again at the next provocation."[58] The foundation of being in a position of learning is first a feeling of safety. The numbers don't tell the story of harshness or the indignities that were part of the paddling.

Jacksonville, Florida, 2015: A teenage high school student is caught running in the cafeteria. Running inside the school is against the rules, so she must be disciplined. She is a Black girl, nearing the age of womanhood. She does not want to be paddled. Regardless, and in need of support for such a physical task, the teacher enlists the girl's male classmates to hold her down while the teacher paddles her. The public paddling was recorded by her fellow students and shared on social media, and local news teams reported the story. Per school policy, at the beginning of the school year, the girl's mother had signed consent and permitted school personnel to paddle her daughter should she misbehave. But, as the girl noted in her interview, nowhere in that contract did it state her male classmates could hold her down while the paddling happened in a public space.[59]

In her book, *Spare the Kids: Why Whupping Children Won't Save Black America*, Stacey Patton says, "The fact is the terrifying damage imposed by slavery and Jim Crow to Black children is now being repeated in Mississippi's all Black districts, where paddling has been institutionalized and continues to be supported by Black parents who sign opt-in forms granting teachers and administrators permission to assault their children's bodies for minor offenses."[60] In Alabama alone, Black males make up 24% of the school population and 35% of the paddled population. While spanking girls is less common in that state, Black females still make up half of the females being paddled, despite being only about 25% of the population. All levels of schools use paddling in Alabama, from the elementary to high school years. The top paddled Alabama school, serving the middle school years, used the discipline technique on 301 of it's 464 students, nearly 65% of that school's population in 2013–14. The top-ranked paddling high school in Alabama reportedly paddled 41% of its students that year.[61]

Educational disparities on test scores and graduation rates are well documented.[62] Black and Brown and poor children do not fare as well as their White and wealthier peers. There are multiple racist and classist mechanisms that support these disparities. While multiple strategies are needed to mend these entrenched disparities, the use of physical punishment and how it is doled out is one starting point. We can't deny the discriminatory perspectives that any adult can carry with them. Some behaviors are problematized on certain students, while ignored on others. Loudness in a Black female might be considered behavior worthy of discipline, while in a White female, it might be considered an annoyance to ignore, and even a sign of potential leadership in a White male student. Behaviors that are labeled as defiant or uppity are based on perspective and are vulnerable to misinterpretation by school personnel— especially when schools are overwhelmed with multiple demands on their time and resources, just like families can be.

But it's even deeper. Black, Brown, and male students are punished more harshly, with stiffer penalties than female and White students. Our inner racism gets to play itself out in sanctioned actions that include activities that would be physical assault in any other setting. Many people, Black and Brown people included, hold oppressive racist notions that assume Black and Brown bodies are stronger than White bodies, that the skin is thicker, that Black and Brown people feel less pain.[63] These unspoken racist notions likely influence the force of the paddle in schools. Males, regardless of skin color, are subject to similar sexist notions of being able to handle the harder paddling. And in a sad account of our understanding of the nested circles, counties with higher levels of explicit racial bias exhibit the greatest school disciplinary disparities.[64] Where the community is more racist, the school corporal punishment is too.

In 2006, eight of the 10 states with the highest incarceration rates were states that allowed school corporal punishment.[65] If a single student was to share the common identities of the children most likely physically punished in schools, they would be male, Black, and have a disability.[66] These tough disciplinary actions are linked to disproportionate numbers of Black and Brown people in the judicial system as adults.[67] And the commonalities and disparities exist across the nation, not just in some parts of the country.[68] The biggest inequality of all lies in the downstream sequelae that manifests similarly to kids who are spanked in their homes. Long-term outcomes on spanked students are harder to identify, partly because of reporting and privacy laws, but the research findings still reveal multiple negative outcomes. Kids paddled in schools, or who receive some form of corporal punishment, most often with a wooden paddle, are more likely to have had lower grade point averages in school, feel less connection to their school community, experience more depression in young adulthood, and carry on the spanking tradition in their own homes, with their own children.[69]

The silence, and hence the quiet acceptance, of school paddling continues. In a policy report on the state of the schools, the silencing of research data on physically hitting children continued. "In 2014, the U.S. Department of Education and the U.S. Department of Justice issued a widely publicized joint report . . . that summarized racial disparities in suspensions and expulsions; no data were presented on corporal punishment, and the only mention of corporal punishment was a brief remark that it has the potential to be used in a discriminatory fashion."[70] Classrooms across the country are microcosms of institutional racism and structural disparities.[71] Dubbed the "school-to-prison pipeline" by the Dignity in Schools Campaign,[72] schools are noted to criminalize Black and Brown children at higher rates than other kids. This pushes kids out of the school system and into the typical problems that follow from a lack of education.

In 2016, the US Secretary of Education, John B. King, wrote a letter to all school districts urging the end of physical punishment in schools. King, a child of public-school teachers, and a previous teacher and principal himself, wrote, "School-sponsored corporal punishment is not only ineffective, it is a harmful practice, and one that disproportionally impacts students of color and students with disabilities. This practice has no place in the public schools of a modern nation."[73]

Paddling Hurts Teachers Too

"Not one accredited teacher college teaches people to paddle," says Paula Flow, director of the Hitting Stops Here campaign and Parents and Teachers Against Violence in Education.[74] Teachers don't want to spank. Teachers enter the profession of education because they care for children's well-being and want to be positive influences in their lives, not because they want to hit them for not behaving well. Very few teachers want to paddle a child, and far more of them are comfortable with detention and removal of privileges.[75] The layers of nested circles provide risks or benefits for teachers too. Teachers and principals who have experienced violence in other areas of their lives, as witnesses or perpetrators, are more likely to perpetuate physical punishment in their school.[76]

Public schools often make considerable efforts to help students feel comfortable to optimize their learning. Enormous amounts of resources are funneled into ending school bullying, and the risks of violence and mass shootings do not seem to be lessening. For teachers and administrators, hitting students, paddling them on the behind, undermines their efforts at relationship building and creating a positive learning environment. "Children have a right to learn without violence, whether in public, private, government, subsidized or religious schools. Safe, respectful, learning environments benefit students, teachers and the wider community."[77]

Teachers and principals who use paddling must deal with their own resulting emotional fallout after the paddling incident, then go home at night to be with their own families; that makes for some intense inner turmoil, as well as a tense learning environment for both students and teachers. Teaching is stressful enough without adding corporal punishment to the pile of responsibilities. This is difficult for administrators too, who are expected to lead the educational institution and set a positive tone for learning. "As the administrator of a high school, I would find it particularly tough to spank someone else's child," said a school superintendent in Florida. "When you see a child cry because of something you've just done to him or her, it's not a pleasant feeling," he said. "To me it's very disturbing."[78]

Efforts to End School Corporal Punishment

In January 2019, a group of congressional leaders introduced the *Ending Corporal Punishment in Schools Act*. The law would have assured that no school that participated in corporal punishment would receive federal funding. One of the original sponsors, the late Alcee Hastings from Florida, stated:

I am pleased to introduce the *Ending Corporal Punishment in Schools Act of 2019*, legislation prohibiting any educational institution that allows school personnel to inflict corporal punishment on students from receiving federal funding. Corporal punishment is an outdated, barbaric, and ineffective practice that has no place in our schools today. Still legal in 19 states, more than 100,000 students were physically punished by being hit, slapped, and spanked at school last year. Corporal punishment is disproportionately used as a form of punishment for African American students, male students, and students with disabilities. The time has come to end this practice once and for all. I look forward to working with my colleagues to ensure the passage of this important legislation to make schools safe places where students can learn free from harm.[79]

The law did not pass. The 20-page bill was updated and reintroduced in 2021, and according to professional sources, was given a 3% chance of passing.[80]

Around the world, 130 countries have banned corporal punishment in schools, while 67 countries allow it.[81] School physical punishment is banned in all of South America, Europe, and large parts of Africa and East Asia. Countries where it is legal in some or all schools include Angola, Indonesia, Myanmar, the United States, India, Guinea, and the Republic of Korea. The list of countries banning school corporal punishment is growing. Sri Lanka in 2021 condemned school corporal punishment, recognizing its roots in colonialism and its contrariness to traditional Sri Lankan culture. Spurred by a court case of a child's permanent hearing loss in one ear from a teacher's hitting, the Sri Lankan Supreme Court stated, "It is unacceptable to consider that a child assaulted may not be entitled to remedy while an adult in the same circumstances would be entitled to such relief."[82]

Safe to Learn is an international initiative aiming to end school physical punishment worldwide and any other form of violence in schools so that children can feel safe to "learn, thrive, and pursue their dreams."[83] The initiative addresses violence between students and aims to stop all forms of violence in schools, including bullying. To end school corporal punishment in the United States, there are a few options. The remaining states can ban the practice through legislation. A federal law could tie federal funding to the elimination of school corporal punishment, requiring an all-out cease on the practice to receive federal education dollars. Or a review of *Ingraham v. Wright* could be reconsidered.[84] A lot has changed since 1977 when the *Ingraham v. Wright* case was heard. Back then, school corporal punishment was not cruel or unusual, but now 31 states, a clear majority, have outlawed it.

Dr. David Gill made the final closing comments during that long debate at the American Psychological Association Convention in 1976. There were no winners in that debate. What he said back then about school corporal punishment is relevant to hitting children in educational settings today:

> If the function of schools and their personnel is to reproduce the prevailing social order, then, I am afraid, corporal punishment is not only desirable but even essential. . . . We must learn to respect authority be it competent or not. We must learn to function in hierarchical organizations, to find a spot for ourselves within such hierarchies, to get ahead within them, to control those below us, and to pay respect to those above us irrespective of their qualifications. There is no better preparation for fitting into such alienating structures than fear of authority figures and oppression of the human mind. And this is what our schools now do. . . .[85]

6

Spanking Around the World

> Societies in which children are hit have cultural norms and beliefs that
> label corporal punishment as different from violence between adults.
> But in reality, the basic elements are almost identical.[1]
>
> —Andero & Stewart

The human baby is the most socially influenced creature on Earth.[2] We teach
our next generation how to live through a slow process of learning, growing,
and adapting to the world around us. Humans, even as babies, can be aggressive, seemingly without teaching or modeling. Normal behaviors of the
human baby from 6 months of age can include a scratch, poke, pull, yank, and
slap, with no intent to hurt. One generous explanation is that toddlers do so
in an eager desire to get to know others. A lot of toddlers bite, and children's
hitting gets harder as they age. Move toward the age of 2 and temper tantrums
with sometimes serious outbursts can begin. A toddler's tantrum can involve
thrashing, screaming, stomping, wailing, and theatrical facial expressions.
After age 3, these kinds of outbursts can escalate to throwing objects and even
hurting oneself or others, and sometimes the child is in such a fit that no effort at reason can work—the child has lost control. Part of parenting toddlers
is helping kids manage their emotions as a way of preparing them for middle
childhood, attending school, and getting along with others. That can seem a
formidable goal when your child is in the midst of a tantrum.

As we do with many human behaviors, we look to our mammalian or primate relatives for similarities and explanations. Mammals invest immense energy, food, and care into raising their young, and among mammals, humans
are the extreme. It takes at least 18 years to guide a human into maturity, and
many would argue that age has extended well into the 20s in modern life. Our
nearest mammalian primates (such as lemurs, monkeys, and apes) take a
long time to mature too, and they share some parenting characteristics with
humans.

Spanked. Christina L. Erickson, Oxford University Press. © Oxford University Press 2022.
DOI: 10.1093/oso/9780197518236.003.0006

Evolution and Spanking

We're not the only animals that hit, and it's such a long part of our ancestral history that we may have evolved this way. Like humans, most primate hitting occurs in the family group rather than among other social relationships.[3] Vervet monkeys, from the mountains of East Africa, have nearly constant contact between mother and baby. Adult monkeys, only weighing about 5 pounds, are trim and cute, with gray fur, black faces, and long tails. Vervet mother and child pairs attach in ways that are familiar to humans, with the mothers holding their infants close to their chest and facing them for long periods of time.[4] For primates and humans, physical punishment is rare for the infant's first year of life.[5] It increases with age, with low levels in infancy rising until 2 years of age when parental hitting peaks for Vervet monkeys, similar to humans. The 2-year-old Vervet is larger, requiring more food and resources. The maternal monkey needs the ever-heavier offspring to transport themselves. When the infant is about 2 years of age, like in a human family, the mother primate often has additional responsibilities that she needs to begin caring for; a sibling is arriving.[6] Conflicts ensue over time with the parent, resources for food, attention, and play. This unavoidable conflict is rooted in the different perspectives of parents and offspring. The offspring wants all it can get from the parents, whereas the parent sees the need to share among existing offspring and future offspring.[7] Conflict ensues, and disciplinary tactics, including hitting, are used as the parent attempts to quickly move the offspring toward independence and utilize fewer parental resources.

Primate researchers note that prime time for monkey physical punishment is when the needs of the parent are most different from the needs of the offspring, almost exclusively related to access to the mother primate, resources, or regulating sibling rivalry.[8] Primate physical punishment is not connected with teaching a lesson about dangerous situations or behavior. As the primate ages, and needs less maternal support, punishment wanes. Evolutionary biologists conclude that primate physical punishment appears more often to support the needs of the parents than the needs of the offspring.[9]

Evolution isn't only a biological process, it also is a social one. Evolutionary baggage, sometimes called historical baggage, is a behavior that sticks despite its usefulness being lost or its purpose long forgotten. In the long span of human history, as societies have matured and developed, humans have moved away from violence across all spheres of society; reductions in mass murders, wars, and violence in prisons, schools, and other social institutions continue to move toward less physical violence.[10] It may seem contrary in a time of heightened access to news from across the globe; however, the longest view of our human existence has shown we drive toward violence-free choices. Slowly, but we do. Things that used to be normal human behaviors would shock us today. It is almost hard to believe how categories that we abhor today were perceived in the past as normal.[11] Previous human behaviors that were acceptable, like gun duels, beating a spouse, and public hangings, are all vestiges of the past, with slivers of existence in modern society that shock us when they occur. Spanking could be a kind of historical baggage we haven't let go of yet, even though it doesn't fit with a contemporary world that generally abhors hitting other people. The future is likely to reflect similarly on our current behaviors. Two or three generations from now people may be shocked at the spanking of today. The record shows that over time we keep moving away from hitting inside the family in all its forms, but the last holdout is spanking.

Humans, more than any other species on Earth, learn to integrate and modulate their emotional, intellectual, and behavioral responses. We call this maturity. It provides us a balance of using our thinking selves and our emotional selves. In the beginning of the parent–child relationship, more emotional responses are used to soothe, calm, and care for a baby, and as children become adolescents there is more integration of thinking and intellect as the parent assists the child to prepare for the complexities of modern adulthood.[12] When our parenting and discipline efforts support what we are becoming, rather than what we have been, we evolve as families and society.

Spanking Worldwide

Worldwide, up to 90% of children experience forms of physical punishment to their bodies.[13] Comparatively, screaming and yelling at children is high worldwide too; at least 75% of families and likely many more participate.[14] Overall, 1.3 billion children, aged 1 to 14, experience punishment to their bodies each year.[15] The rates may be even higher because forms of physical punishment that are considered typical, like spanking, are underreported. In a study of nine countries, it was found that 67% of girls and 72% of boys experienced physical punishments in their home in the past month. Ten percent of these punishments were physically severe[16]. Also worldwide is the experience of sadness, fear, pain, shame, and guilt that children experience because of the hitting.[17] Similar to other studies, the number of parents who believed hitting a child was necessary to raise them was smaller than the number of parents who had actually used a form of hitting.[18] Globally, parents find themselves hitting kids, whether they believe in physical punishment or not.[19]

Around the world, there are various interpretations of the usefulness and right of a parent to hit their children. The perspective on childhood, the roles expected of parents, history, culture, and religious beliefs all influence how a country creates social guidelines and laws that address the tension of parents' rights to discipline versus the protection of children from parental harm. The way families show love and affection, if and how they deal with conflict and pursue work and education, and how they teach their children are all expressed differently across societies and cultures.

An international definition of child abuse from the United Nations (UN) Convention on the Rights of the Child states: "intentional use of physical force or power, threatened or actual, against a child, by an individual or group that either results in or has a high likelihood of resulting in actual or potential harm to the child's health, survival, development or dignity."[20] The UN language, developed for the whole world, is challenging to operationalize universally, so legal language and family, cultural, and professional interpretations vary.[21] While spanking may seem to have a universal definition, how children are viewed, the roles of parents, understandings of discipline, and even the words used to describe spanking shape the meaning of hitting a child. In the United States, we tend to view the behavior of children through the lens of *good* or *bad*, and other cultures may accept behaviors as simply those of children.[22] The justification for and implementation of spanking change by community and culture and are likely not universally shared by people around the world.

But there are some constants. Physical punishment is common, found in nearly all societies. Research on spanking shows that those same negative outcomes—aggression, intimate partner violence, depression, and substance abuse—are increased for spanked people all over the world.[23] Where there is greater inequality between men and women, there is more family violence, including more physical punishment of children.[24] Societies that accept hitting a partner, most often a female spouse, are more accepting of hitting children. Internationally, women who believed husbands were justified in hitting their wives were more likely to believe physical punishment is necessary in child-rearing. These women were also more likely to report that their child had been violently disciplined in the home in the past month. Women who did not believe a husband was justified in hitting their wives had a lower acceptance of hitting children.[25] Societies with more power inequalities, such as stratification based on wealth, gender, or race, can be indicators of physical punishment. The researchers for one study explain:

> If parents want children to fit into a society with inequalities in power, might parents choose corporal punishment to convey dramatically that some people are

much more powerful than others? After all, to a child, parents are clearly powerful, not only are they taller and physically stronger, they also control and dispense important resources. So perhaps parents think, consciously or unconsciously, that corporal punishment is a dramatic way to convey the discrepancy in power between themselves and their children and that the perception of this discrepancy by the child will generalize to an acceptance of power inequalities later on when the child grows up.[26]

While spanking may be universal, what is considered worthy of a spanking is culture bound.[27] Some cultures believe that any show of disrespect to an elder is worth a smack, where another culture may find the behavior must be far more egregious to warrant a hit of any kind. How we judge others' spanking is connected to our understanding of their intention. If the parents' intentions are considered good within that culture, people tend to accept those spankings with less judgment.[28] If a culture believes parents are always right, and hitting is for learning, then the culture will support spanking. But the cultural practices can support other options too. Countries who discipline children without hitting them show good outcomes from their culture's sanctioned discipline methods with children.[29] Spanking is not the only option, and it does not have to be the last resort. The research on spanking holds true wherever you go in the world. The negative outcomes from spanking are experienced by children everywhere. So even if the adults in the culture are more accepting of spanking, the negative outcomes persist.[30]

Four young people in British Columbia, Canada, went to Parliament Hill to debate the right of children to spank their parents and teachers. Citing adult mistakes like drunk driving and ignoring bullying in the classroom, the debaters suggested spanking could be an option for adult punishment, doled out, of course, by the youths themselves. Absurd? That was the point. The youths were protesting Canada's law that allows "reasonable force" in spanking by a parent, teacher, or another caregiver.[31] Canada's law allows spanking between ages 2 and 12, minus objects, anger, and degradation.[32] Reasonable force, the youth demonstrators claimed, was being misused by adults. It often justified spanking that seriously hurt children. Repealing the Canadian spanking law doesn't mean police will interfere after an occasional smack on the bum in the grocery store. "That is not what we want to see," said one youth, adding, "I think it's not realistic to see a 180-degree turn on how children are disciplined overnight."[33]

Canada provides a good example of the complexity of trying to figure out what is allowable in physical punishment and what is maltreatment. Laws set parameters to help legal and medical professionals determine abuse, and laws act as a guide to help parents determine whether they should spank, and if so, how hard. In Canada a spanked child must be between ages 2 and 12 and have the intellectual capacity to learn from a hitting. The force used must be minor and without objects. The head can never be hit, and the hitting must never be the result of parental emotional turmoil such as loss of temper or frustration. The child must never feel degraded. If you spank within these limits, it is considered "reasonable force." Trouble is, studies in Canada have shown that abusive parental punishment fell well within all these parameters, meaning that many parental acts of child abuse can actually be justified by law.[34] Wherever we go in the world, the research findings remain. The most reliable predictor of child abuse is physical punishment.

Women and Children

I loved Elvis Presley movies as a kid. One weekend, I thought it would be fun to watch his 1962 blockbuster *Blue Hawaii* with my daughters for a fun family movie night. It was winter and the escapism of music and beaches seemed appealing. Until the spanking scene. In one of those beautiful beach scenes, Elvis grabs his budding love interest, pulls her face down over his lap and spanks her. She kicks and screams, and he lets her know this is her for own good. Shocked at the sight of a grown man hitting a woman, and with my daughters watching with me, I quickly fast-forwarded the movie. How had I not remembered that scene as a child in the 1970s? Probably because the spanking of women was normalized in that film and many others. John Wayne and Lucille Ball had spanking scenes too. From the 1920s onward there are dozens of movie scenes of adult women being hit on the buttocks, often over the lap of an adult man.[35] The men and women in these films were often in romantic relationships, and the hitting combined words of love or expressions of attraction along with demands and authority. I didn't remember the Elvis spanking scene because it wasn't unusual in my growing up years. Spanking of adult women was, unfortunately, not relegated only to the film reel.

Stories of spanking have also shown up in social relationships in which a man shows a woman that she has made a mistake. This overlay of presumptive power is essential to the spanking experience. The exposure of the buttocks, not facing the spanker so as to be unable to respond, is a submissive and vulnerable position to be in. It is literally coming up from behind. Women throughout the ages have suffered at the hands of men who have sometimes created crimes specific to women so that punishment, often flogging on the buttocks, could occur.[36] Witchcraft and other "crimes" ascribed to women who were then "punished" by paddling the buttocks. Working class and poor women were especially vulnerable to false accusations or recriminations if they did not perform their work well enough. But it happened across economic spheres and even into professional workplaces.

It was a Saturday morning in the newsroom of a city newspaper in Alabama in 1973. Twenty-two years old at the time, and just beginning her career, Veronica Pike Kennedy was called into the office of her 40-year-old boss, H. Brandt Ayers, to review some pieces for publication. He asked her to read him some of his work, and as the conversation about the piece ensued, Ayers told Kennedy she was "bad" and stated, "Do you know what I do to bad girls? I spank them." Ayers forced Kennedy over a desk and spanked her 18 times with a newspaper ruler. Across the expansive newsroom, another young reporter in his 20s witnessed the spanking. Veronica kept the experience quiet, not wanting to stain her budding journalistic career. Thirty years after the incident, Ayers, the owner and chairman of a chain of newspapers, admitted to this spanking, and others of his female employees. Ayers stated that a doctor had told him to use the technique to "calm" women down.[37]

In 2019 a female news reporter was on the sidelines of a running race in Savannah, Georgia. Speaking live on camera, you can see the elated runners coming up behind her, many of them waving and cheering, thrilled they are nearing the end of a challenging race. In clear view, a man, who appears to be old enough to be her father, runs up behind her and slaps the news reporter on the ass. The reporter is stunned for a few seconds, loses her words, and then continues to report her story. He spanked her. A one-swat public spanking. Change the gender of the reporter, and one can clearly see that the spank would likely never have happened. The runner was charged with sexual battery and was banned from related athletic activities in the area.[38]

The spanking of children and the spanking of women are only shades of gray in difference from each other in relation to power and dominance. Since the 1980s we have known that where there is hitting between spouses, there is more hitting of the children.[39] Sometimes, what is considered discipline worthy, especially physical discipline, are reinforcers of cultural stereotypes of what it means to be male or female. Spanking has been used on girls and women to reinforce their submission to authority, often to male figures, who attempt to control how they behave.[40] Connecting violence against women to childhood punishment is a case made by the Committee on the Elimination of Discrimination Against Women, citing young girls as worthy of protection too. "When a woman is assaulted by a family member in her own home, her human rights are violated; when a girl is physically punished by her parents in her own home her human rights are violated."[41] Children today are in the position adult women were in decades ago. Children can be hit by the most important people in their lives, without impunity, until it crosses into abuse or maltreatment, too late to prevent trauma, abuse, or even death.

Rights of Children

Women's rights and children's rights are very closely connected. Women are the primary caregivers of children, and most societies still hold them most responsible for the well-being of their children. When we move beyond research or a God-granted belief in physical punishment, the human rights of children who are hit is a fundamental concern. Rights of children to feel safe in a home free of physical threat, rights of parents to care for their offspring, the right to privacy of the family, and the right of the government to intervene when a child is in danger are all connected. Before the late 1800s in the United States, there were no laws protecting children from abusive parents. A full 100 years later, in 1989, the UN, with help from such organizations as Amnesty International, created and adopted a human rights treaty, called the Convention on the Rights of the Child. It was one of the first international documents to include statements on social and cultural rights along with political and civil rights. Every country ratified the Convention on the Rights of the Child—except for the United States.[42] In paragraph 29, the Convention on the Rights of the Child identifies "harmful practices," one of which is physical punishment.[43]

Forty-nine years after the 1945 Convention on Human Rights that focused on adults, this special convention on children declared a belief and offered a legal extension to children as human beings and rights-holders. As rights-holders, children are entitled to the same protection of human rights as any adult. Children too should be free from the worry of assault or physical punishment, and living free from violence is at the heart of the Convention on the Rights of the Child.[44] Children have a right to be free from "any punishment in which physical force is used and intended to cause some degree of pain or discomfort, however light."[45] The Convention identifies society's moral obligation to provide dignity and protection for children's growth and development. It is a government's responsibility to assure rights are upheld, generally through law. The UN Convention rejects any suggestion that spanking is fundamentally useful for parents or children, even if culturally the hitting has been justified. Physical punishment of children always violates children's rights, making culture bound exceptions moot.[46]

Any punishment using physical force intended to cause pain or even discomfort, as well as any that is cruel and degrading, is considered a violation of children's moral right to respect, human dignity, and physical integrity. Beyond this moral argument, physical punishment is a legal violation of children's right to equal protection under the law, due only to their status as children. When social norms support hitting a child, moral arguments are often used to challenge spanking. When we evaluate spanking through a moral lens, we tend to view spanking as harmful no matter the intentions of the parent or the mistake of the child.[47] The moral lens overrides our intentions to include culture and context, and instead hinges on the larger universal agreement that showing force through hitting is wrong for anyone, anywhere. A position in which physical punishment of children is permitted in a society, yet child abuse is forbidden, is untenable.[48]

Maybe you're wondering, what is that UN thing again? It's the worldwide organization of countries, aimed at peace, health, development, and humanitarian assistance around the globe. The UN provides a forum for countries around the world to engage in dialogue, share perspectives, and work on solving complex problems together. It is the team meeting of the world, and part of their strategic plan is to end violence against children worldwide. You may be thinking childhood violence refers to things like trafficking, abuse, living in a war zone, big stuff. Those are included, but family violence counts too, and just like people wouldn't tolerate people being hit by their spouses inside the privacy of their home, many people don't tolerate kids being hit by their parents in the privacy of their home.

It's important to understand that the Universal Declaration of Human Rights is not legally binding on a government; it includes statements of fundamental freedoms to aspire to. Countries who are members of the UN are obliged to move toward ending physical punishment in recognition of the Convention on the Rights of the Child. The process of transforming society's view of children, to seeing them as holders of human rights and ensuring they cannot be hit and hurt in the guise of discipline, is a process that takes time.[49] As explained in the *International Journal of Pediatrics*, "Children being hit and hurt by those stronger and more powerful than them reflects the inequality and discrimination in relationships that are the very building blocks of violent societies and the very opposite of what it really means to respect girls and boys as individual people and holders of human rights."[50] More than half of all UN member governments are committed to ending the physical punishment of children.[51]

The US has never ratified the Convention on the Rights of the Child. With no commitment, the rights of children remain suggestions, ideas, or concepts to consider with no legal mandate to uphold them. Nonetheless, a human rights perspective makes any argument for physical punishment indefensible. Determining acceptable hitting from abusive hitting is an impossible task, sustaining and maintaining such a distinction is untenable, and the costs of missed calculations are simply too great. Children throughout the world often have the lowest status in society. Spanking is often used as a way to humble children, make them willing to learn. Such humiliation is never or rarely given to, nor deemed acceptable for, adults.[52] Recognizing that a child can be victimized, like an adult, is a step toward ending spanking, a form of discrimination allowable only because of age.[53]

Spanking Outlawed

The worldwide effort to end physical punishment of children is well established and growing. While it currently has a nearly imperceptible presence in the United States, ending physical punishment has a strong foothold in many nations around the world. The movement started in the 1970s, and the pace is undeniably constant. Sweden, in 1979, was the first country in the world to ban all forms of physical punishment of children in all settings, including spanking in the privacy of the home. After Sweden's ban of hitting children in 1979, it took 10 years for only two other countries to do the same. But by 1999 the number of countries banning spanking rose to eight, and by 2009 that number had risen to 24.

As of 2022, 63 countries have banned all forms of physical punishment, including all forms of spanking, swatting, whupping, smacking, and other hitting tactics parents use to correct or discipline. Nearly all of South America, much of Europe, a handful of countries in Africa, Greenland, Mongolia, Japan, Turkmenistan, Nepal, and New Zealand have banned physical punishment of children in any setting. In these countries it is illegal to spank in the home, paddle in school, or intentionally physically hurt a child for learning or discipline, even if you are the parent and even if you do not leave a bruise or injury.

When Sweden banned hitting in 1979, they coupled it with a nationwide communication and information campaign to parents and children. They delivered a brochure to every household in the country and posted signs on milk cartons, and within 2 years it was estimated that 90% of Swedish citizens were aware of the new law. While Sweden did have an increase in referrals to child protective services, they did not have an increase in prosecution of child maltreatment.[54] At the time of the ban, about 50% of parents spanked their children in Sweden. The acceptance and use of spanking fell to about 30% in the 1980s and reduced to only a few percent after 2000. Poland saw similar drops in acceptance of spanking. Their ban occurred in 2010, and hitting children fell by 32% over the next 8 years.[55] Making something illegal doesn't stop all humans from participating in the behavior. Countries that ban spanking must still enact child abuse laws, investigate reports of abuse, and protect children from parental maltreatment.

In most countries where spanking is banned, the efforts at law reform are an attempt to hold parents responsible, not in a criminal way, but rather through methods to change the families' response to disciplinary issues.[56] The laws are not meant to separate families or criminalize parents, but instead to help maintain family integrity by building new methods of parenting practices. Legally banning spanking won't stop it completely. A cultural shift is required.[57] That usually takes outreach, public education, and lots of conversation to help individual families begin to determine new options. April 30 is International Spank Out Day.[58] Started in 1998, the goal is to end all physical punishment of children. Over generations, changing norms and awareness efforts like Spank Out Day have slowly moved the parenting options from allowance of any and all physical punishment to protection of children. The global community is not stopping there. There is a robust movement to protect children from physical punishment in all spheres of their life.[59] The effort is not to create an overreaching government with a presence inside the privacy of the home. The legal mandate expects to bolster a new social consensus that spanking children, even in the privacy of your home out of love, is unacceptable. It builds a rationale that hitting our partners is domestic violence, hitting our pets is animal cruelty, hitting our children is child abuse. The legal structure doesn't stop hitting overnight, but it supports incremental change toward parenting without hitting.

Legal language banning corporal punishment sheds light on the culture of the country and expectations of families. The following are some samples of the legal language in nations where spanking is outlawed:

Poland, Banned in 2010

Persons exercising parental care, or alternative care over a minor are forbidden to use corporal punishment, inflict psychological suffering and use any other forms of child humiliation.

Honduras, Banned in 2013

It is prohibited for parents and every person charged with the care, upbringing, education, treatment and monitoring of children and adolescents, whether in a temporary or permanent basis, to use physical punishment or any type of humiliating, degrading, cruel or inhumane treatment as a form of correction or discipline of children or adolescents.

Nepal, Banned in 2018

Corporal punishment is prohibited in the home . . . and [this] prohibits all corporal punishment of children, who are defined as persons. . . . Each child has a right to be protected against all types of physical or mental violence and punishment, neglect, inhumane behaviour, gender based or discriminatory abuse, sexual abuse, and exploitation committed by his/her father, mother, other family members or guardian, teacher or any other person. . . . [G]iving physical or mental punishment or disrespectful behavior in home, school or any other setting is criminalized as a form of violence against children. . . .

Japan, Banned in 2020

A person who exercises parental authority over a child shall not discipline the child by inflicting corporal punishment upon him/her or by taking other forms of action that go beyond the scope necessary for the care and education of the child. . . .

There are a few countries where no prohibitions on physical punishment to children exist—the rarest legal standing. In Africa, these countries include Botswana, Mauritania, Chad, Nigeria, United Republic of Tanzania, and Somalia; in the Middle East, Saudi Arabia; and in the Far East, Malaysia. This means that children can be spanked at home or at school, or by another parental proxy or caregiver. Other physical punishment is allowed as well, often determined by cultural acceptance of practices. In these countries the broad cultural acceptance of hitting children upholds parents' rights to do so.

The Global Initiative to End All Corporal Punishment of Children is an international organization supporting and tracking the movement of laws and efforts to protect children from physical punishments. Their goal is to ban hitting of children in all settings worldwide by 2030, in line with the Sustainable Development Goals of the United Nations.[60] The reason? They believe a ban on physically punishing children will lead to world peace. They believe what Gandhi said: "If we are to reach real peace in this world, and if we are to carry on a real war against war, we shall have to begin with the children."[61] The idea that peace starts with one person and flows outward toward the rest of the world and influences the nested circles—they take that seriously. The Global Initiative literature states, "Ending violent punishment is key not only to ending violence against children, but to reducing violence across the whole of society in the longer term. Violence against children is the foundation and source of much violence in society."[62]

There is evidence to back them up. Countries that have banned physical punishment of children experience fewer youth physical fighting events.[63] The international group Global Partnership to End Violence Against Children has worked with countries around the world to accelerate efforts to end physical punishment in all forms. These countries—Armenia, El Salvador, Indonesia, Jamaica, Mexico, Mongolia, Montenegro, Nigeria, Paraguay, Philippines, Romania, South Africa, Sweden, Sri Lanka, Tanzania, and Uganda—are actively studying rates of physical punishment of children, instituting legal language to ban the practice, and making efforts to educate their citizenry on the changes. Members of this Global Partnership tailor outreach efforts to their cultural and geographic heritage and share new options as exemplars in instituting change across their social institutions, including families.[64] Banning corporal punishment generally evolves from banning hitting and paddling in childcare, residential settings, schools, and juvenile justice settings before banning physical punishment in the home, the place of last resort.

The reason these organizations believe that ending spanking can bring world peace is not as far out as it sounds. Experts in conflict note that the "shape of conflict" is the same between individuals, communities, and nations. It is only the scale that is different.[65] If we understand spanking as a show of force at the familial level, we can see that show of force represented in our community and at an international level. The nested circles. Violence prevention experts want to reduce violence in all spheres, including the ones in the family, which is the first place in which we experience any form of violence.[66] But they are working against a common belief system. Those who believe physical punishment is a necessary parenting practice tend to believe that physical child abuse is less widespread than it is.[67] We can open our eyes to a larger understanding. If hitting one's children is illegal, it will be like giving a vaccine, a dose of stopping abuse before it starts. If the spanking never happens, you effectively stop the chance for maltreatment. The vaccine worked. No risk, only protection.

There is likely no legal area murkier than the rights of parents to raise children as they believe, coupled with the equally strong belief that a community should intervene when a child is in danger. But if we focus only on individual family rights, we shroud the social sanctioning of hitting. No one person is responsible for the harm that is caused in spanking; it is a structural behavior, meaning it is integrated and accepted seamlessly across social structures. In the United States, more parents have supported the right to physically punish their children than those who support a child's right not to be hit.[68] It is accepted because of the structure of society that supports it; you can hit this singular person if you are the parent and the child is 17 or younger. Without that structure, it is assault. The mother of a 10-year-old boy shared the contradictory feelings best when she said, "I think anybody should have the right, however old, not to be hit around the head or smacked or physically abused in any way. But I also think that if I need to get through to them and nothing else is working . . . I ought to be able to smack them to get the point across. So, yes, it's very contradictory, but I still think both of them, if you know what I mean."[69] Parents are unwitting victims of this structural violence. The social sanctioning of hitting kids, combined with the knowledge that any other hitting is assault, leaves parents in a conundrum. These structures that are invisible to parents encourage them to physically hurt the people they love most and, in the end, to hurt themselves too.

The Right Side of History

Private family life is in the midst of democratization. We are relearning what are participation and leadership and patterns of interaction for a happy family life. Shere Hite wrote in 1994 in her book, *The Hite Report on the Family: Growing Up Under Patriarchy*, about a process that is continuing today: "[T]he extreme aggression we see in society is not so much a characteristic of biological 'human nature' (as Freud concluded), nor a result of hormones. Rather, it is brought about by the way in which power and love are combined in the family structure: in order to receive love most children have to humiliate themselves over and over again before power."[70] As always, the behaviors of our private realm of home life will affect our public spheres. We have the knowledge and even the duty to make our private family lives more skilled at problem-solving and better at using language so that we can improve our own lives and extend those skills into the nested circles.[71]

For large parts of the world, where physical punishment of children is banned, spanking is an absurdity. When absurdities are expressed by the masses, the absurdity is normalized. Alice Miller noted that which is monstrous has a seed in what is normalized.[72] Scientific and philosophical experts on violence agree. The violence of home is connected to the violence of the streets, and of the school, and of the workplace. Spanking and whupping are simply part of a "well-oiled" hitting machinery[73] that causes us to undermine our most important relationships, advantages our weakness rather than our strengths, and teaches others to normalize harm to the human body. This violence-making machine is worldwide, with seeds in families that sprout in neighborhoods, ride the bus to school and the subway to work, and grow into community strategies to control and demand and penalize and fire, and criminalize, and hate.

Ending physical punishment of children will exert influence on other forms of violence in society; a pressure of nonacceptance of all forms of hitting other people. Stacy Patton writes in *Spare the Kids: Why Whupping Won't Save Black America*: "We must also ask how punishment shapes our consciousness and our conviction about authority and power, about the ways the coercive domination so many people experience becomes the authoritarianism that pervades American life and politics."[74] Truly, in a time in which we do not accept overt racism, sexism, and homophobia, our acceptance of this form of ageism is contrary to our general abhorrence of denying human rights. Indeed, the most fundamental of rights is to simply have human rights.[75]

Human behavior is often counter to the efforts of law, educational bodies, and expert institutional advice. Humans continue to quietly spank our children, despite negative research findings and a wide arc of organizations and national bodies who either disparage or outlaw spanking. But there is a growing sense of a false dichotomy, one that legitimates, in an arbitrary way, spanking under the guise of discipline and other family hitting as abuse. Dichotomies like these have shown an ever-shrinking pattern throughout history. The giant chasm of child abuse on one end of a continuum and spanking on the other is a steady march toward an ever-narrowing funnel of what is acceptable as punishment.

PART III

PART II.

7

In the Privacy of the Home

There was an old woman who lived in a shoe.
She had so many children she knew not what to do.
So she gave them some broth without any bread;
then whipped them all soundly and sent them to bed.

—English Nursery Rhyme

In the privacy of the family home, without the outside world watching, is where the most life-shaping spanking occurs. Many people don't talk about their current spanking practices; a story from long ago might be shared, but last night's family discipline tactics are likely off-limits. However, occasionally, unwittingly, private family events find a public stage.

In 2018, physician and California State Assemblyman Joaquin Arambula was arrested for charges of willful cruelty to a child, a misdemeanor child abuse charge, when his 7-year-old daughter told her schoolteacher about the disciplinary experience the night before. As Arambula and his wife explained in their public statement,[1] the evening before had been a difficult one as the family tried to settle into their nightly routine. In a moment of feeling overwhelmed, Arambula said he spanked his daughter to discipline her for something she had done, something he'd normally only do as a last resort. As his wife Elizabeth stated, their daughter was angry about the spanking and was still angry when she went to school the next day. All teachers are mandated reporters to child protective services for child abuse, even suspected abuse. So when Arambula's daughter told the teacher about the previous night's experience, the teacher had no other option but to report the incident to local child protective services. What the teacher heard or saw that required them to make the report to child protective services is confidential. What the police chief said is that Arambula's daughter had injuries that were not typical of spanking.

In an act of public education, the police chief is quoted in the *Sacramento Bee*: "It is important for people to know that when you discipline a child, and spank them on the buttocks it is perfectly allowable by law. However, when the level of discipline rises to the level of injury, then that is a violation of the

Spanked. Christina L. Erickson, Oxford University Press. © Oxford University Press 2022.
DOI: 10.1093/oso/9780197518236.003.0007

law."[2] The official charges against Arambula were cited as "cruelty to a child by willfully inflicting unjustifiable physical pain or mental suffering."[3] In his statement, looking sheepish and regretful, Assemblyman Arambula identified himself as a medical doctor, in addition to being a state Assemblyman, and described himself as a healer, and that he is not one to hurt others. His wife was supportive in their efforts to explain the situation. Dr. Arambula stated, "Everyone who knows us in the community and has seen us in the community knows that I am a loving father. I care about my daughters deeply. And I'm just going through a process and trying the best I can to be a husband and father who's putting us back together again."[4] Dr. Arambula was found not guilty and acquitted of all charges.[5]

The private experiences of the Arambula family that night are likely common. What's different is the national attention their family received. Arambula's charge of abusing a child is serious and cannot be taken lightly. But if what the parents say is true, the Arambula family had a typical difficulty that a lot of parents can relate to. They wanted their child to comply with their family evening routines, such as getting ready for bed, and difficulties ensued. The Arambula family story is one that plays out in small towns and big cities wherever families reside, as parents make daily decisions on disciplining their child.

Spanking Disagreements

The police chief in the Arambula story, as he educated about how to spank, attempted to convey that legally, a parent can easily cross over into child abuse. How to spank a child appropriately is a long-standing dispute. Should the parent be a calm disciplinarian enforcing rules without emotion, or is the frustration and anger in the moment key to making the spanking a useful learning experience?

Disagreements on how to spank aren't just a national debate but an internal family debate. Polarities exist within families, creating a point of parenting conflict regarding tactics used or even degrees of difference in force. Even if both parents believe in spanking a child when needed, it may not be in the same ways, with the same intensity, or even for the same offense. How does one negotiate or intervene in the privacy of their own home, the spanking of their child by the other parent, a stepparent, or even a dating partner?

The earliest references to this debate, *Spank Kindly and Never Angrily*, was a textbook used in classes for parents in Wisconsin in 1927. "The most excellent spanking process has fallen into disrepute because so many parents spanked only in anger. This is harmful. . . . Be a judge, calmly enforcing a sentence justified by domestic judicial procedure."[6] By the 1970s the pendulum had swung in the other direction. Fitzhugh Dodson, in his plain-speaking book, *How to Parent,* noted that children can cause strong emotional reactions in parents, and advised giving in to these frustrations. "We get fed up when our kids misbehave and we lose our cool and swat them. But that's nothing to feel guilty about. We feel better and they feel better, the air is cleared."[7] Dodson continues, "But if you feel you have blown your stack, it's important to admit it to your child. Above all, don't pretend to him that the sole reason you spanked him was for his benefit. That's as phony as a three dollar bill, and he will know it. The main purpose of spanking, although most parents don't like to admit it, is to relieve the parent's feelings of frustration."[8]

Hitting, in all relationships, is an act of aggression, and so to hit in anger seems a natural option—people do not hit other people when they are calm, empathic, caring, or teaching. In disciplinary moments, parents are not granted the role of learner, only the enforcer. How can a parent manage their frustration and anger for their own growth and development in problem-solving—not just for relief? Can a parent even manage the hair-splitting difference between a legal spanking and abuse in a challenging disciplinary moment? In 1977 an article titled, *Only Spank When You're Angry,* advised, "After all, whether necessary or not, a spanking does mean a small loss of temper or control, and if enough time has elapsed for full reason to take over, there probably are better ways to handle the anger."[9] A 1980 article states, "You sometimes hear it recommended that you never spank a child in anger but wait until you have cooled off. That seems unnatural. It takes a pretty grim parent to whip a child when the anger is gone."[10]

In a National Public Radio Conversation on the topic in 2008, one mom stated, "I strike when angry and only then do it a couple of times and it's got to be with my bare hands so I feel it too so I don't go crazy. But I don't believe in the, 'you must be calm and rational and think it through.'"[11]

For co-parents who disagree on discipline methods, one may hand over the important role of discipline to the other and observe rather than intervene. Within families, there can be assumptions and divisions of belief. One parent may have more influence on parenting. If that parent chooses to spank, the other parent may acquiesce. A parent, who may not believe in spanking, may accept the physical discipline by telling themselves that other families have it worse or that the spanking parent is good in other ways. And so the spanking continues, even within families that may feel unsure if spanking is the best option for them. For the parent who watches or is aware of the spanking, the child can hold the same feelings toward them as the parent who spanks.[12] Observing or even being aware of the spanking is sanctioning, representing parental agreement to the child. The nonspanking parent may rebuff complaints or requests for comfort from the child to be in solidarity with the spanking parent.

In modern times parents seek out social media to find information on their spanking disagreements. On a Christian parenting blog, a parent asks, "Is it normal for my 5 year old son to wet his pants while he is getting a spanking? My son does this whenever my husband or I spank him, but he wets more frequently and worse when my husband spanks him." The moderator responds with a suggestion to have the child use the bathroom before each spanking and queries, "Sounds like he is scared?" But fellow readers' comments show the polarization of people's opinions on spanking.[13] Another reader adds, "Spank him harder for peeing himself, that's what I would do." Followed by another: "If I started hitting you because, let's see, you didn't do something correctly you might wet your pants too. Think about it . . . take parenting classes." Some parents want kids to *fear* the consequences they will dole out, in hopes of keeping kids from acting naughty.

Parental Perceptions of Children

Parents develop early perspectives about their child that are not necessarily logical. A calm and quiet dad may find himself with a hyperactive and aggressive toddler, while the other parent considers the same child energetic and expressive. Parents' description of their baby's temperament can be more related more to their perceptions than the actual behavior of the baby, setting up patterns for interaction early in the relationship. These perceptions are often unknown to the parents; they may go as far back as a conception or birth story that makes the child either difficult or blessed. If we could ask a baby, they might state that there are also difficult parents. For babies, emotional availability from a parent would be comforting, and emotional distance would be stressful.[14]

With these early perceptions, the shared parent–child relationship has begun. Many parents don't see that these first perceptions shape the narrative of their children's lives even at this early age. Importantly, different perceptions and even different measurements are used on kids in the same family. Siblings elicit different responses from the same parents; each is raised in different ways within the same family.[15] Children first discover what kind of a person they are and how they feel about themselves through the reactions of their parents.[16] Children have no choice, they must survive in the family they have, and that is what children do, they adapt. There is no grievance procedure for kids who'd like to make a complaint about their parents. There is one line of authority, and it is through the parents.

These parental perceptions influence the evolving parent–child relationship. It is often difficult for parents to set aside beliefs of how a child ought to be and accept a child as a unique individual because most parents have preconceived notions of what their child will be like. When a child misbehaves, parents may perceive the momentary behaviors as representative of who the child is becoming, frightening parents into responding harshly. Negative explanations for a child's behavior reduce a parent's sensitivity and responsiveness to their child.[17] The child understands themselves through the eyes of the parent and lives up to these perceptions. These patterns become part of family lore and create labels for children that can be difficult to shed, even as adults.

When parents label kids with words like bad, naughty, mean, uppity, rude, lazy, or irresponsible, it affects how the child views themselves and how the parent views the child. If behavior is assumed to come from within the child, then the intervention is to fix that child. If the explanation comes from the situation the child is in, then the intervention is to fix the situation the child is in. Imagine a parent has a son who has misbehaved many times. The parent thinks of him as naughty and worries about taking him out in public because he may misbehave again. The parent is primed to see what they already know about the child: the pattern of bad behavior. When the child behaves well, it slides by unnoticed. Humans make these inferences automatically.[18] If we think our child naughty, we assume he is often up to naughty activities or at least scheming to do so. As parents interpret their children's behavior, they often make a critical mistake. They underestimate the importance of the context surrounding the child and assume flaws in the child. *He did it again; I knew I couldn't trust her; I should have known he'd screw up.* Adults commonly amplify a small human characteristic to explain situations and deflate any contextual explanation. This is called the "fundamental attribution error."[19]

This common flaw of the fundamental attribution error sets parents up for trouble. The perceived difficulty of the child, rather than the situation, encourages parental use of spanking rather than another form of problem-solving.[20] When parents attribute their child's negative behavior as personal to the child's intentions, they are angrier, they are more irritated and ashamed, and their discipline is more harsh.[21] It is the child's behavior that provokes discipline, but the choice of spanking, the force, and the number of hits are influenced by the parent's emotional state and perception of their child. What the fundamental attribution error blinds parents to is that human behavior is largely driven by situational factors, and influencing these external factors can have big effects on kids' behavior.[22]

Parents may need to admit the measurement tools we use on our children are not always realistic. In *Choosing Happiness*, Stephanie Dowrick writes: "We compare our children's progress using measures more suitable for the workplace than the classroom."[23] Parents sometimes expect kids to sacrifice joy, spontaneity, and even learning skills like cooperation to assuage parental fears of future failures. Sometimes the concern is more for the parent's reputation than the child's. Some children are easier to raise than others, some respond more quickly to parental requests, and some find ways to manage themselves and their emotions better. The variety that can live inside one family is as vast as in the entire society. Each child requires us to be a unique parent to them.

Internal Stress

The overarching aim of parenting is to teach children how to mature as individuals in a complex world, but most parents feel their child is a reflection of them too. Successful, grown children are the stuff of parents' dreams. Having expectations about a child's future, abilities, and even potential occupations, long before the child is an adult, is common. This imagination of the social climb of our children is part of the normal dreams and hopes of parents. Imagine your son, a first pick in the NBA draft, and the speech of gratitude for his parents keeping him on the right path. Or imagine your child accepted to that elite college, appreciative of the high standards their parents expected. One can imagine the disappointment felt when kids struggle too. Parenting comes with a whole lot at stake, not just for the child but also for the parent. The potential pride or shame raises parents' anxiety, they may feel they have their child's future on the line, a reflection of their success. Parents may reason that spanking is in response to the severity of the child's misbehavior, but this hides their own internalized stress about their child. "[W]hen a parent hits a child for committing the very infractions that adults have failed to master, they are beating out of their child the negative parts of themselves that they are ashamed of."[24] That stress may be from the child's behavior, or just as likely from the parents' own challenged skills or fear of an unsuccessful child.

Parenting is complicated; that there are thousands of books on the topic is testament to this truth. The stress and fear of a misbehaving child can motivate parents to discipline rigorously. In *Love and Anger: The Parental Dilemma*, Nancy Samalin writes, "All parents harbor a hope that, once their children understand the reasons behind the rules, they will become cooperative. But people, and that includes children, don't always do what they know is best for them."[25] The strong-willed or spirited child will test parental limits in ways that are unimaginable to people who have not been there. A child or family may also have challenges, raising the stakes of doing parenting right and keeping the child from serious problems like school failure, inability to make friends, or delinquency. Pressures to do parenting right and have a child you can be proud of can lead to self-induced and internal stress for parents.

Parenting stress is at least in part related to the never-ending nature of the role. Parental burnout is a real thing and can lead to deep emotional exhaustion that triggers other feelings beyond impatience, to rage or despair.[26] In their book, *Burnout: The Secret to Unlocking the Stress Cycle,* the Nagoski sisters describe parenting burnout as the recognition of the time it takes to get something done, the drain of managing your child's emotions along with your own, the constant reasoning and instruction, the reminders, and the never-ending repetition.[27] This stress can cause a parent to feel short-tempered. Parents don't just feel short-wired, they are, and it can lead to parenting that is neglectful and even violent.[28]

Some of this stress is of our own making, including how we talk to ourselves about our own parenting. When I became a first-time parent at age 32, I was sure I was going to do quite well at the job. After years of fertility challenges, adopting our daughter was a joyous experience. I had just started a PhD program, and I was quite certain I would be a modern mom, managing to advance my education with the new demands of parenting our daughter. It didn't take long for reality to set in, and I realized I was not the mother I had imagined in my years of dreaming about parenting. My certainty that I could do it better faded with piles of laundry, a messy house, lack of sleep, quickly assembled meals, and a realization that I did not have my own time. I hadn't realized how much I needed that. My internal tape of negative self-talk offered me little room for adjustment, empathy, seeing the many good things I did, or even just a break. I had heard of postpartum depression, but my daughter was adopted; I didn't have hormonal changes to blame this on. What I slowly became aware of is that I am a normal mom and judged myself too harshly. My baby daughter was delightful. Smiley, sweet, pretty, easy to please. It was me I was disappointed with. This was a personal transition, and I wasn't as successful as I imagined. The comparison of the mother I imagined I would be to my lived reality was intense, but all in my own head. I finally had to see it as harmful, and intentionally reduce the negative messaging I was giving myself. Sometimes, maybe often, the worst judgments we make about ourselves, or our children, are ideas of our own making.

This kind of internal stress can wear on parental temperaments. Any parent can identify with the range of emotions that a child can elicit in them. The change from relative calm to complete joy to absolute frustration is different for each parent, but the quickness of it can surprise many. Inside the privacy of the home, children's temperaments interact with parental personalities in complex ways. It is possible to dearly love and loathe a child. Bonnie Harris, in her book, *When Your Kids Push Your Buttons and What You Can Do About It*, says, "Allow yourself to be brutally honest. You are not alone in having monstrous thoughts about yourself or your child."[29] Children themselves can be an enormous stressor and can trigger parental behaviors that may surprise a parent—to love them so deeply, yet at the same time to feel shame in their behaviors, who they are, and even who they might become is a complex emotional roller coaster. And parents need to know that those who find parenting stressful are more likely to spank.[30]

We can't blame kids for the punishment we give them, but to say they do not play a part isn't true either. Acknowledging the role of children in increasing parental stress is not to blame them[31] but instead to offer insight to stressed parents. Children are spanked for various misbehaviors, and parents may feel uncertain or unaware of strategies to improve kids' behavior. The most challenging misbehaviors are hardest for parents to successfully address. Kids who fail to pick up their clothes or engage in other common childhood misdeeds are less likely to be spanked than kids who commit an act that violates another person's "rights," like taking a toy or being aggressive to another person.[32] These kinds of moments call for our most complex parenting skills. Parents can feel intense stress when their feelings toward their child or the role of parenting don't match their ideas of what a good parent should be and how a good parent should feel or act.[33] Some parents are exasperated by their child's immaturity. Depressed parents spank more, and parents caught in a spanking cycle might feel more depressed. Having a challenging parenting experience can be distressing, and feeling that your parenting skills are not up to task can also be depressing. Parents want to parent well, and feeling like a failure at the most important job in the world is a setup for low confidence and high anxiety.

Even usually well-behaved children can ignite assumptions and bring on emotions causing unexpected parental actions. Children often save their most emotional and provocative behavior to try out in the safe environment of home. Privacy of the home allows children a safe space to express their wide range of emotions and allows parents to respond with discipline they may have never imagined. If parents are fueled by feelings of powerlessness and even catastrophizing thoughts, they will discipline more out of fear of losing control over their child than what the infraction deserves. Sometimes, parents lose control of themselves.

Parental feelings are internal, but they have an outward manifestation, one that is a form of communication, whether we realize it or not. When a parent pays attention, they'll feel physical manifestations of their internal feelings while parenting. They might furrow their brow, scowl, raise their voice, breath heavier, and stomp around before the spanking begins. This was all setting in the day I was in the kitchen and my kids started arguing in the living room, but I failed to notice my own physiological changes because I was too busy thinking what naughty kids *they* were. Denying the range of potential feelings good parents can feel leaves us less able to protect our child from ourselves when necessary.[34] As a 1946 parenting book warned, "In all disciplinary situations the adult must keep an eye on himself as well as on the child. He should feel certain that he is not demanding too much. . . ."[35] And kids are aware. Children as young as age 4 have reasoned judgments about parental disciplinary tactics, including recognizing fairness and even abuse.[36]

External Stress

Parents may be demeaned by a boss or coworker, underappreciated for their efforts, relied on by too many people, talked to angrily at a store, flicked off on the highway, feel stung by a social media post. Feelings like these are often held in until a safe place is found, and that is usually home. The desire for parents to hit their children can be influenced by their daily life experiences. Parents justify spanking children for the child's behavior but may be blinded to the external stressors that create their frustration and impatience. A kid's resistance to parental requests can feel like one more challenge to a parent's self-esteem and respect, already threatened by experiences in the outside world.[37]

A child behaving badly may induce parental frustration, but the parent's own stress over work issues or other problems can be the hidden inducer of spanking. The child's behavior does bring on the spanking, but the parent's stress and emotional overload is the real reason for the punishment. Sometimes parents are simply exhausted and overwhelmed. In *The Mother Dance*, Harriet Lerner writes, "We may be stir crazy, on the edge of violence, or exhausted, or sick, or depressed, or otherwise needing to put ourselves first."[38] This exhaustion can lead to impulsively using the easiest parenting tools we have. For generations that has been spanking. Impulsive spankings are one of the hardest reactions to change.[39] Partly because the venting of the frustration can be reinforcing to the parent. The child quiets down, the parent feels some catharsis, and in the moment it seems successful.[40] But the long-term impacts of impulsive spanking cannot yet be felt by the parents, and the immediate relief will not outweigh the long-term consequences.[41] When parents are burdened with concerns, they don't always have the mental and emotional resources available to be the kind of parent they want to be. Stressed out parents can be overly sensitive to their children's negative behavior, even if in the range of normal. In hopes of ending perceived misbehavior quickly, parents respond harshly. These methods leave no space for reasoning, discussion, repair, or emotional support.

Uncertainty and shame can stifle the sharing of spanking experiences. Kids intuitively know that discipline practices, especially those that include hitting, are not something to be talked about. Yet, the personal realm of the family is connected to society. Parents raise children to go out into the world and participate in school, arts and sports, and wider family and community activities. Families provide a "linking function"; they explain the obligations and opportunities of the wider world, and this links a child's personal identity to a social role.[42] Each family interacts with the world around them in ways unique to them. What is sometimes beyond awareness is that parents' concerns about how their children will be perceived outside the home influence the disciplinary choices inside the home. External pressure to parent children who will bring pride to the family, rather than shame, is a powerful motivator for many parents, and it shapes discipline.

Our fears about the outside world influencing our children can encourage us to spank. When a Black parent explains to their children how to behave in a world with racism, they are linking their family life to the racism their children will face in society. Parents may believe that not to spank early is to risk their child's future. "My father was so very afraid. I felt it in the sting of his black leather belt, which he applied with more anxiety than anger, my father who beat me as if someone might steal me away, because that is exactly what was happening all around us."[43] Ta-Nehisi Coates in *Between the World and Me* suggests that sometimes our parents, who love us the most, are afraid for us the most. A parent who may see a world around the child that may hurt him, may hope to punish that child into safety. Its seed is love, even if misplaced. Looking at his child and realizing that he can beat him or the police will, Coates writes, " I understood the cable wires, the extension cords, the ritual switch. Black people love their children with a kind of obsession. You are all we have, and you come to us endangered."[44] Spanking seems like the right answer to safeguard children in a world ready to harm them, but the actions are based in responding to fear rather than bravely creating something new. Resmaa Menakem, a somatic therapist and social worker, suggests that the impulse to spank to keep our children safe can be reconstructed into building resiliency into our children, our families, and our communities.[45]

Parents can feel intense anger at their child, a new kind of frustration they may have never experienced before. With this strong emotion, it seems a parent should *do* something. So when the parent acts on the anger, they may later feel intense guilt for the feelings they had and the actions they took. If we parcel out the feeling and recognize it as normal and not something regrettable, our actions may change. In *Love and Anger: The Parental Dilemma*, Samalin states: "Our goal then, is not to eliminate the feelings of anger from our parental repertoire. We couldn't, even if we wanted to. Rather, it is to find ways to express ourselves when we are angry that do not hurt, insult, demean, or inspire revenge and rage in our children."[46] When we do this with our kids, we learn to express frustration and anger in healthier ways. It leads to different options for problem-solving. Our growing skills as parents spill over into other parts of our lives.

Cycles of Circular Causality

I was hanging out at the park with my kids one afternoon. There were just a few families there, and it was dusk, not long before the kids would be heading off to bed. Two little boys, brothers about 5 and 6, were playing on swings not far from where I was. Soon they started fighting over a particular swing.

"I want a turn!" said the 6-year-old boy.

The 5-year-old swung happily and refused to comply with his older brother's request. The older boy continued, "C'mon, give me a turn." And when that didn't work, he demanded, "You've had enough time, get off!"

Their father was at the park too, and had been attentive enough, but was distracted by his phone. Finally, the younger boy on the swing kicked his older brother in the stomach, who quickly responded by pushing his little brother off the swing. That's when dad looked up and saw the last few seconds of the brewing spat. He marched over, gave the older brother a quick spank on the behind, took him for a time out, and the younger brother got back up on the swing, triumphant. Had Dad looked up mere seconds earlier, he would have seen a different story; the little brother likely would have been spanked and hauled off.

Who is naughty sometimes depends on when you enter the story. The problem with physical punishment is not just that the punishment might not work, it might even backfire. A parent may be punishing a specific child but fail to see the larger problem situated in a set of interactions, not the individual child. If one child is frequently punished for joint problems, that child may begin to see themselves as the source of the relationship problems, building resentment toward a legitimate unfairness that the parent does not see. This is the reason I banned the "F" word with my kids. I'd attempt to intervene in a sibling squabble only to hear two viable explanations of whose "fault" it was. In a moment of clarity, I hollered at my daughters, "No more F-word! There is no fault, it's just a problem!" That led to simply moving forward, leaving blame behind.

These cycles of behavior occur unwittingly in all families and can have another common pattern. Imagine Dad at home with his child, happily playing. Mom comes home from work, and great joy ensues. Child and mom greet each other, hug, and share a few moments of connection. Mom and Dad then begin to talk, recounting their day and addressing the needs for the evening's events. The child, completely removed now from either parent's attention, begins to misbehave. It works. Both parents now communicate with him by reprimanding; it is negative, but they are giving attention. So the child continues to misbehave in similar ways. Mom and Dad start cooking dinner. One of them gets a phone call, and they are distracted from the child who now really misbehaves, and a spanking ensues. The real seed of the problem? A cycle of seeking love and attention, in small interactions, with the child attempting to secure their place in the family. In *Conflict Theory of Corporal Punishment*, the author states, "Punishment is sometimes interpreted in psychodynamic accounts as a sign of love. . . . [I]t is not so much a symbolic displacement as an immediate gratification of the demand for attention. Better negative attention than no attention at all."[47] From the child's perspective, as they ramp up the negative behavior, the parental attention comes back, inadvertently reinforcing their negative behaviors. The child's behavior is an "extreme form" of attention-seeking, and even though unpleasant, it is preferable to being ignored.[48] Some have suggested parents rename the negatively attributed behavior of "attention-seeking" to "connection-seeking."

As these cycles become ingrained in family life, they become nearly invisible. The previous experience encourages a quick analysis of the next incident, often leading to the same conclusion. When siblings fight it is usually a particular child's fault, or a parent rationalizes, "This child always acts up as soon as I need to get something done!" If spanking is part of this cycle, it can escalate from a smack on the behind when young, to a slap in the face, to a full-on brawl in the teenage years. In these cycles the spanking may be covering up a worse problem: a lack of connection. The attention and energy given to the child's negative behavior may be the most intense parental connections the child gets. Couple this with a lack of attention when children behave well, and it is a perfect setup for continued misbehavior and missed chances for positive parent–child interactions.

Kids see patterns and dynamics in the family that parents don't. They have a unique view from their angle in the family. They are aware, way more than parents ever know, of subtle differences that suggest inequities in parental love and acceptance. In *The Mother Dance*, Harriet Lerner writes, "Kids have an amazingly strong sense of justice in family matters, and they will notice the most subtle inequalities, such as the fact that a parent always laughs harder at their brother's jokes or seems more sympathetic with their sister's disappointments."[49] No parent can see all the contributions to the problem; they're not all visible. So parental intentions can be lopsided by parents unable to see the full picture of the family dynamic.

When these behaviors develop into repetitive patterns of interaction, they become cycles of circular causality, and the parent–child dynamics reinforce each other without awareness. Many parents will tell you that kids don't comply with requests until they know a parent is serious about it. This pattern develops through repeated cycles between the child and parent. When a parent requests an action but doesn't actively follow through, the child learns they don't have to respond—yet. This can escalate from talking into yelling and sometimes hitting. A cycle of circular causality ensues, on repeat and in overdrive, and the parent and child don't even know they are on it. The real danger is that the ratcheting up of anger makes the chances of overly harsh discipline more likely. Over time, the cycle often intensifies rather than weakens, and if not interrupted these unhealthy relationship cycles follow us into adulthood.

All families end up with cycles of circular causality; the trick for parents is to make sure they are healthy and beneficial cycles. Parenting shapes us, and it can be for the better. Active parental attention toward positive child behavior is one of the most powerful parenting tools we have. The cycle is just as powerful in the positive realm. When kids begin to display progress in things like reading skills or kind and thoughtful behavior, parents increase their investments in them, even in material ways, such as time and activities that benefit the child.[50] When we nurture kids' positive behavior, our kids help to bring out good parental behaviors, setting up a positive and healthy cycle of circular causality. If we are intentional about it, parenting can make us better people.

It is not selfish to want to be a parent in a way that encourages your growth as a human being. It may seem counterintuitive at first to do things that are in the best interest of the parent. But the best interest of the parent likely has positive ramifications for the child and family culture too. A parent who struggles with conflict resolution at work would behoove themselves to try out conflict negotiations with their children. Practice on your 5- and 7-year-old, ramp up your skills of influence and negotiation, and see how good you can be without your work colleagues watching. Can you engage them? Practice having the right words for your audience, use the right tone of voice, carry yourself with confidence, choose the most descriptive words you can, and see how your kids respond. Ask your kids to grade you and tell you what you can improve on, encouraging them to engage in fixing the problem.

Parent–child relationships are power-laden, dynamic relationships that change as the child grows. Adapting these healthy cycles to the age of the child is one of the most enriching aspects of parenting. Each new year brings a child closer to their own sense of adult power, and the parent must begin to withdraw their power over the child. In all parent–child relationships, the power of the parent erodes as the power of the child increases, as a natural consequence of the move toward independence. Conflict can occur when this usually slow shift accelerates or stalls. Even with careful attention, maintaining a healthy cycle of circular causality between parent and child can be a challenge. The patterns, the contexts, and the occasions for obedience inevitably change with age. It is in the moment-to-moment experiences that we build or degrade our relationships. It's not just the big things but also the million little things that add up over time. Over these years, there are few things more stabilizing and safeguarding than genuine affection and respect between parent and child.[51]

8

In the Public Sphere

> According to the ruling of Judge Austin of Indianapolis, parents have
> a legal, as well as moral right to spank their children at any time of the
> day or night, and no matter how much outsiders are annoyed by the
> wails of the punished child they have no redress.[1]
>
> —*Journal of Education*, 1908

The Complete Observer

Bruce Brown covertly observed parents and their children in public places
from 1976 to 1978. He's not a creeper, he's a sociologist. He used a sociological
research method called the "complete observer." This method required him
to not involve himself or interact with those being observed. In fact, the goal
was for people to not know they were being observed. He wanted to understand and document the discipline of children in public places. Brown went to
a shopping mall weekly. He watched and made notes on all the parent–child
interactions he saw. People at malls know they can be observed; they are aware
there are others around. Pick your nose? You can do that at the mall, but you
might get some awful looks from others. Brown knew that people are unlikely
to display publicly behaviors they prefer others not know about.[2]

Brown sat, watched, and took copious notes while at the mall. He watched
and wrote about kids misbehaving and what parents did about it. A recurrent
finding was that children were being disciplined for not "fitting in" while in
public. Kids were in adult spaces, and they weren't acting like adults. All the
parents, with children of different ages and genders, utilized what he called
"restrictive techniques." They hit, yelled, or gave direct commands. Brown
observed that children not acting like adults threatened the parents' presentation of themselves as good parents, causing embarrassment and distress. If the
child is flawed, the parent is too. This potential sense of shame explained the
parenting techniques used in the mall as parents hoped for quick results in the
management of their child's misbehavior. Brown concluded that until parents'
own sense of self-esteem can be separated from their children, they will not

Spanked. Christina L. Erickson, Oxford University Press. © Oxford University Press 2022.
DOI: 10.1093/oso/9780197518236.003.0008

be able to use less restrictive or demanding parenting techniques in public. It seems at first glance that the measurement of a successful outing to the mall is a well-behaved child, but if we cling to that outcome alone, we miss out. The point isn't perfect children, but rather little people learning how to figure out different environments and how to act when in them.

In 2020 at a mall myself, face masks required, I saw a mom struggle with a child not walking fast enough, lollygagging some might say. Clearly frustrated, she hit her child's bottom and then dragged him by the arm as they emerged from a department store. It's a fairly common sight, much like the one written about in a Texas editorial. Two little girls, ages 2 and 5, were unusually rowdy while shopping in a store with their mom. Maybe they were running around the aisles, playing tag between racks, or begging for things they weren't allowed to have. Likely their behaviors drowned out their mother's requests to settle down. They left the store and before settling them in the car, the mom spanked each of them for their misbehavior. A woman in a nearby car saw the incident and started yelling, following the family, waving her arms. The mother and girls pulled over to hear: "You're going to jail for beating your kids, you're going to jail!" the woman shrieked. Unperturbed, the mother of the two girls spat "Shut up!" out her open window and headed home. When she recounted the story to her husband, he wrote an editorial to his local newspaper, "Does this lady know where she is? In some places in America, a parent might face trouble for spanking their children. But this is Texas. We do things a little differently here. In fact, spanking is not only legal in Texas, many in law enforcement encourage it." He felt the matter was not for others to involve themselves in. He stated in his editorial, "I spank my children because I love them. No matter what one thinks or how often they say it, spanking a child is not abuse. In fact, in my opinion, spanking a child is responsible parenting. Parents who choose not to spank their children are hurting their children more than helping them."[3]

Strict or Permissive

One accusation nonhitting parents face is that they are overly permissive. Parents who do not punish children physically sometimes fear reprisal and judgment by other parents. In a small study of nonspankers, these parents described a sense of feeling deviant to the wider culture and a desire to hide the fact that they do not spank their children. Rather than claiming a nonspanking position, they were more likely to simply say that their child was not naughty enough to deserve one yet. Interestingly, when their children's behaviors were described, they were equivalent to the behaviors of children who had been spanked.[4] For some, there is a misconception that parents who don't spank don't discipline their children at all.[5] Parents who choose not to spank may have to deal with peer pressure suggesting they are too weak to discipline their child firmly, spoiling them, or even accusations of not loving them enough to parent with assertiveness because *withholding* a good hard spanking is sometimes believed to have negative outcomes for a child.[6]

This supposed requirement of spanking has infuriated other parents into believing they should hit other people's kids for them. In public places, parental behaviors that look like spoiling or ignoring sometimes occur in an effort to distract or at least delay a tantrum or other misbehavior. In searches on Facebook using the word "spank" or "whup," I came across advice about spanking other people's kids, and suggestions for parents who don't spank that they should start. In one post a male parent suggested that a "stronger parent," even if a stranger, knows when a "bratty-ass" child needs to be corrected, and the stronger parent should be legally allowed to walk over to another parent, take off their belt or shoe, and spank that child. In a similar post, a photograph shows a man sitting at the end of his driveway with a sign that says, "Free ass whoopin's," and he holds a wooden paddle. This belief that spanking is a requirement for misbehavior is so strong some adults act on them, even with other people's children.

A 2-year-old boy and his father were standing in line at a grocery store. The child wanted candy and pleaded and whined to get some. The father ignored him. A man standing in line behind them was tired of hearing the child cry and whine as he begged his father to purchase the candy. Feeling the child needed discipline, the man grabbed the boy by the arm, swung him around and spanked him two times. The father was stunned. The police were called, and the man was arrested and charged with child battery and obstruction.[7] The father stated he doesn't spank his kids, "That's my son and at the end of the day I'll discipline him how I believe he needs to be disciplined." Had the father spanked the child himself, there would have likely been no criminal charges.

Shame and Love

Taking kids to shopping malls and restaurants gives no privacy for parenting efforts. Parenting in public is stressful, especially when trying to complete adult tasks, like renewing a license, attending an appointment, going to the bank, or anything that requires decision-making. Failing to respond to misbehaving children in public can lead to public scrutiny; responding too harshly can lead to public outcry.

When there are few children in a public space, a parent with young children can feel out of place. Not all public venues are welcoming to kids, and it doesn't take long for a parent to find a young child distracted without warning. Each place they enter is a new environment to explore, and parents who feel their children are less able to stay on task and follow directions can find themselves wanting to use spanking more frequently.[8] Most adults adjust their behavior depending on the context. Young children don't have that ability yet. Bringing children out in public makes parents hyperaware of their child's behaviors. "So many parents in my groups talk about the tremendous pressure they feel from their own parents, in-laws, friends, the media or the elusive 'they' to parent in the ways they are struggling to leave behind. Parents feel scrutinized by the eyes of the world telling them they are either disciplining too much or not enough. If children misbehave in public, parents feel humiliated and blamed. It is no wonder we feel so responsible for our children and try desperately to control their behavior."[9]

Even being at a playground can be stressful. Ever had your kid push another child? Bite them? The shame you feel and the impulse to discipline them so others know you are handling the situation can be a powerful motivator.[10] Parents know they are being observed, and the watchful gaze of family and friends, even strangers, affects the way the parent responds. A parent displaying irritation and distress at controlling their child can exacerbate the child's emotional and behavioral response in a negative way. Kids can read us, even at age 4 a child can reliably identify parent hostility and determine what is abusive discipline or not.[11] Kids may not respond in ways parents expect with their efforts at control.[12] How welcoming the public space is to children and the parent's own sense of confidence and self-esteem influence the response of the parent. At that moment, with others watching, parents may want to raise their sense of power and assure others they have authority over the child.

On the outside, parents may look to be powerful in the relationship, but the public display often veils feelings of powerlessness. Those parents working the hardest to gain some power over their child may actually feel they have the least. They may feel shame in the behaviors of their child and respond in ways that surprise even the parent. As one parent noted, "People look at me like I'm some kind of ogre when I discipline her in public. I'm to the point where I just want to avoid a scene at all costs. . . ."[13] Even small amounts of criticism can make parents defensive; add on feelings of insecurity and self-doubt and you have the recipe for unsure parenting. A misbehaving child in a public setting can bring on a cascade of shame. In her book on shame and vulnerability, *Daring Greatly: How the Courage to be Vulnerable Transforms the Way*

We Live, Love, Parent and Lead, fellow social worker Brenee Brown points out that when we are the most judgmental and self-righteous is when we have the greatest levels of uncertainty. "When I feel shame, I'm like a crazy person. I do stuff and say stuff I would normally never do or say" and "parenting is a shame and judgement minefield precisely because most of us are wading through uncertainty and self-doubt when it comes to raising our children."[14] Our own fear and anxiety for shame seduces us into believing we can have clear answers to our parenting dilemmas. Parenthood is a major source of dignity in an adult's life. Feeling judged for being inadequate, or failing to discipline one's children, can be a major impetus to believe you should do something—and spanking is the easiest thing to grab on to.

Many parents believe they want the best for their children, but they have an unspoken agenda to have successful children to fulfill their own sense of self-worth. This can set any parent up for trouble, especially if they hold very high standards with a narrow definition of what is successful—a combination impossible to fulfill.[15] Public shame shrinks our ability to be present in the moment and consider what is best for our kids, and makes us resort to responding to what is best for our self-esteem. One of the best ways to dissipate shame is to respect honest feelings. On a National Public Radio show, a storyteller commented on his parenting experience. As he and other parents stood in line for a bouncy castle, they shared parenting stories. As one parent noted, no one ever really tells you how hard parenting is going to be, or that you sometimes won't even like your child.[16] Separating our sense of self-esteem from the behaviors of our child is one antidote to shame-induced parenting. "Our whole job is provide, protect, love and facilitate. It's not to own . . . it's not about us," said Dwyane Wade in his interview on *The Daily Show* about parenting his teenager.[17]

Public Interventions

It was sunny out, and four of us met at a local park for lunch in the middle of the workday. Each of us had grabbed a sandwich from a local deli or had packed one from home. It felt so good to catch up with colleagues and friends, chat about our lives, and take a break from the challenging work we do. We were all women, three social workers and a teacher, all with graduate degrees, all with young children. As conversations often do with fellow parents, we started telling stories about our kids. They ranged from hilarious antics to exasperating parenting moments. One story stood out to me, and while I can't remember the specific acts of the child, I have never forgotten his punishment.

One mom, a social worker, tentatively shared that her 7-year-old son was so naughty she had to "put tabasco sauce in his mouth for swearing, spank him and ground him." She shook her head and laughed, in a kind of "What else could I do?" kind of way. We all nodded, empathizing with her struggle and mild embarrassment, and even laughed along with her to lighten the mood. Another mom followed up with a story of her brother getting the same punishment years ago. We each understood the struggles of discipline, and we all knew she was a good and loving mom. But I went back to my office and couldn't shake the story, the complicity of us all sanctioning the hitting. All four of us care deeply about children's well-being, that's why we chose the professions we did. Yet we laughed off an uncomfortable hitting and tabasco sauce story that seemed hard for my friend to share and likely hard for her son to bear.

Any respectable professional will confront child abuse. But spanking has rarely been considered a form of maltreatment. Couple that with the desire to respect family privacy, and having a conversation with others about their spanking practices can feel pretty dicey. We need tools, a platform, a reason to have the conversation. It would help if those conversations happened in multiple locations, like faith communities, neighborhood groups, parent groups, and medical visits. For many parents, one of their trusted relationships for parenting advice is with their pediatrician. Like any workplace, pediatric clinics are made up of people with diverse opinions on spanking.[18] Seventy-eight percent of pediatricians believe spanking is a poor disciplinary technique, and most pediatricians are aware of the negative outcomes found in research. Simultaneously, 90% of pediatric patients' families feel there are unmet needs in parenting guidance during their clinic visits.[19] Advice about responding to children's negative behavior is complex and hard to get to in a clinic visit that covers so many other topics and includes a wiggly and possibly uncooperative child. Giving tools to have these conversations can reduce pediatricians' discomfort in talking about spanking; it reduces their positive attitudes toward spanking too.[20]

To help identify parents struggling with discipline, Seth Scholer, a pediatrician at Vanderbilt University, developed a Quick Parenting Assessment. It starts with the question, "In the past month, what have YOU done when your child needed to be disciplined?" Options include redirecting; taking away a privilege; threatening to spank, smack, pop, or slap; following through on the spank, smack, pop, or slap; or angrily raising your voice. Depending on the score of the questionnaire, parents are divided into risk categories. Low-risk parents are commended for their positive parenting, and medium- and high-risk parents are given a prescription to the Play Nicely program.[21]

Play Nicely is a descriptive title. Pediatricians and preschool teachers from the National Association for the Education of Young Children and psychologists from the American Psychological Association developed the multimedia learning tool that asks the parent, "What would you do if your child hit another child?" and walks through options for responses. Parents are coached on choices as they move through the program. If they choose a hitting technique, they get a prompt that cues them on the problems associated with spanking or slapping and offers alternatives. It works. Most parents who used Play Nicely reduced their positive attitudes toward spanking.[22]

Still, parents need to see what is in it for them, and they should. Adam Zolotor, a physician out of the University of North Carolina at Chapel Hill, suggests asking parents during a clinic visit, "What are you feeling when you spank your child?" and "How do you feel after you've hit or spanked your child?" Parents take notice; they discover that swatting kids happens when the adult doesn't feel good or is having negative thoughts about their child. Many feel guilty afterward, ruminate on the scenario, worry, and take those sad and frustrated feelings with them into the next social encounter with partners, kids, work, and neighbors.[23]

It makes sense that when professionals, like pediatricians, support physical punishment, the parents they work with are more favorable to physical punishment too.[24] The American Academy of Pediatrics had encouraged parents not to spank, but in 2018 that stance changed, and got much clearer. "The American Academy of Pediatrics opposes striking a child for any reason. Spanking is never recommended." Also, "If a spanking is spontaneous, parents should calmly explain later why they did it, the specific behavior that provoked it, and how angry they felt. They might also apologize to their child for their loss of control. This usually helps the youngster to understand and accept the spanking, and it models for the child how to remediate a wrong."[25]

For the most part, we don't involve ourselves in the behaviors of others in public; sometimes, people don't intervene even when it's necessary. Unless we feel a compelling ethical or safety reason to act, we allow people to behave as they wish. But fear for a child's safety is a powerful motivator that can spark people to intervene in a public place. Thirty-seven people who had confronted a parent disciplining their child at a shopping mall, waiting for public transit, or some other public place were interviewed to understand their reasons for intervening and how they felt afterward. All the people felt compelled to act because they were bothered by the style and manner of what the adult did to the child for punishment.[26] They felt the parent acted unjustly and that the child was victimized rather than disciplined. They felt they were meddling in other people's business, and their lack of expertise or authority made them question themselves. Many regretted portions of what they said. Most felt they could have been more succinct, more empathic, or less emotional in their response. They feared making it worse for the child by angering or embarrassing the parent. It was clear that a public intervention by a stranger was not a receptive time for any parent to reflect on their parenting. In the end, the people who intervened felt their concern of child abuse justified their actions.[27]

When parents feel they have limited value, especially in a certain community or public place, they attempt to control their children's behavior with extreme parenting measures. Parents' efforts to make their children behave are often a response to the unspoken rejection of them in that public place. Empathy may be the answer. The moment-by-moment recognition of reality and acceptance of it is advocated by Byron Katie in her book, *A Thousand Names for Joy*. She describes her response to public displays of parent–child stress: "If I see a mother hitting her child, for example, I don't stand by and let it happen, yet I don't lecture the mother. She is innocently acting from a belief system she hasn't questioned. Because she believes her stressful thoughts, 'the child is disrespectful, he isn't listening, he shouldn't talk back, he shouldn't have done what he did, he needs to be forced into submission,' she has to strike out." Katie states that love and empathy is what allows us to intervene, and that love must include the *parent* and child.[28]

Being empathic is a novel way to intervene in a potential public disciplinary moment. Rather than feeling like you have to be a hero and protect a child or admonish a parent who you think is parenting incorrectly, empathy focuses on engaging in a neutral way, with understanding. Parents have different styles of parenting, and respecting parents is one of the most important parts of intervening in public.[29] Offering a knowing smile, commenting on how taking kids shopping can be tough, or noting how you've been there with your own kids can make a world of difference for a struggling parent.[30] The Minnesota Children's Museum hired "funstigators," people whose sole job is to distract children out of their bad behavior and defuse any chance of a negative parent–child interaction while waiting in line for tickets. Parents attempting to complete adult-centered tasks provide enough minutes for a young child to notice the loss of parental attention and engage in behaviors to get that attention back. While funstigators appear to focus on the kids, the greater goal is to give parents time to take care of check-in and purchasing tickets. You can see the relief as the impending meltdown dissipates when the funstigator steps up. And the effort is believed to offer reverberations into home life. As parents return home from public places with kids, they are not carrying the anger and shameful memory of a child's tantrum that stretched their parental limits and might incite more frustration at home.

Empathic responses and funstigators hope to reach folks before they ever have a brush with uncomfortable public parenting situations. Making a space more comfortable for children and their parents can be part of design: building design, room design, process design. Nearly all public places are made for adults, and few are designed with intergenerationality in mind. Ramps aren't just for wheelchairs; they work for strollers too. Offering a play space, or a chair next to a computer for a child to sit, and some materials for coloring are all options that can be used to dissolve, and even prevent, parent–child stress in public places. Those little kid grocery carts are more than just cute. They help prevent negative harried shopping experiences. The goal is to be the parents' ally and offer supportive and welcoming family spaces. The larger goals of happy families and pleasant experiences increases the protective factors and decreases the risk factors in the nested circles of all people. Influencing one circle in the nest will have reverberations across other circles in the nest. If violence can spread between the nests, then kindness and successful problem-solving can too. Deciding to spank or not is a decision not just for the child but also for the parent, the family, and the community.

Nested Circles

Each of us influences the nested circles we live in and the nested circles of others. Families have protective factors and risk factors in their immediate nests, and from nests farther away too. The effects from the outer nests are just harder to see. Through physical punishment, violence starts early in life, but as children grow, it becomes part of a continuum of violent experiences.[31] Families and the communities they live in often share similar risks and protective factors. Cultures that condone mild forms of violence, such as hitting children for punishment inside the family home, are more violent overall at the community level.[32] If you live in a neighborhood with violence and crime outside your family's home, you might think it's possible to close off the world and create a peaceful family unit shielding your loved ones from these social problems. But you can't, not completely.

Neighborhood conditions offer protective and risk factors for youth. Even little children, just 3 to 5 years old, and in families who infrequently spank, had increased childhood aggression living in a neighborhood with high crime and violence.[33] The qualities of the neighborhoods, towns, and countries we live in affect our nested circles and encourage parents and children to behave in certain ways. What happens in the world outside our homes influences what happens inside our family home.

Privileged families have an often-unrecognized freedom to make mistakes in social graces in public and not be judged or punished for them. In the insightful public-school documentary, *Love Them First: Lessons From Lucy Laney Elementary,* set in an economically poor community, the school principal ponders the children she just saw at the coffee shop on her way to work. She notices that the middle-class and White families have more freedom to spill their beverage or play loudly; no one chastises them or threatens to kick them out. She is disheartened, knowing children of color, especially poor children of color, could never feel so comfortable behaving like that inside a public space.[34] Economically poor Black and Brown children experience shame and judgment in public in profound and subtle ways that privileged children don't. This often compels parents of color to keep their children close and demand they are on their best behavior to protect them from the judgment and disgrace they may be subjected to for even typical childhood antics.

Some people's nested circles are filled with privileges like permanent homes, good schools and parks, steady employment, and loving family members. Some are filled with disadvantages like poor-quality housing, struggling schools, lack of green space, inconsistent employers, and stress-filled family members. Every nested circle has advantages and disadvantages, and the balance is different for everyone.[35] Families with many advantages buoy their losses and shield their struggles. Families with many disadvantages have fewer anchors to hold onto and struggle to protect themselves from life's burdens. Parents living in nested circles with lots of advantages have more leverage for punishments. Low-wealth families have fewer opportunities to modify social and material experiences as a form of discipline or as a form of reward.[36]

For all of us, our nests are built on connected relationships between these nested layers, doling us each out doses of protections or privileges and risks or oppressions. Figuring out our unique individual response to this doling out of life's benefits and burdens through the nested circles is what we call life. Being spanked inside a nested circle full of protective factors may be different from being spanked inside nested circles heavy with risks and burdens. But that doesn't change the reverberations between the nests. When our nested circles contain any kind of violence, we are more likely to experience it in another layer of the nest, either as a perpetrator or a victim.[37] We spread what we know, whether we are aware or not.

9

Modern Family

> The question isn't so much, "Are you parenting the right way?" as it is:
> "Are you the adult that you want your child to grow up to be?"[1]
>
> —Brenee Brown

Bad Moms. No, I don't mean your neighbor or sister-in-law. The 2016 movie. It poked fun at the stress and pressures of momhood, the constant judgment and comparisons, the idea that there is one right way to raise children. The movie follows three friends as they struggle with their public persona of parenthood compared with how they really feel about parenting. "We have to bring down the perfect moms!" is their rallying cry as they toast their plans to rebel against the expectations of culinary-style lunches, well-behaved children, and a magazine-cover home life. As they wallow in their stress at a local bar, they malign modern parenting.

> "Do you know what I hate? There are so many fucking rules now."
> "Yes, God. Don't punish your kids."
> "Don't say no to your kids."

The movie pokes at expectations for families, many of them unwritten and handed across contemporary cohorts with emphasis on perfection and competition. Modern parents can be pretty passionate about their kids. Spanking appears to have such a quick reward for a busy parent. The swat with a stern "no" can be a relief for parents who are juggling multiple kids, carpools, and activities, along with their own adult lives involving careers and relationships. No wonder spanking has lasted so long.

Modern Parenting

Raising a child is infinitely complicated and is made more so by the rate of change in the world around us. Each generation of parents has a new world

Spanked. Christina L. Erickson, Oxford University Press. © Oxford University Press 2022.
DOI: 10.1093/oso/9780197518236.003.0009

to raise their children in, so different from the world they were raised in.² Traditionally, parenting has relied heavily on a hierarchy. Those in power know more than those below them, held together with a belief system that there is a right way to behave in the world. The role of the parent in the hierarchy is to teach that right way; it is the most loving thing to do. Modern parenting stretches into more egalitarian forms of parenting, in which parents nurture their children's values and encourage earlier critical thinking. Buoyed by broader cultural change of equality and expanding education, modern parenting practices are a reflection of this egalitarianism. In most societies, physical punishment fades as egalitarianism rises.³ This doesn't mean parents and children have equal power. They can't; parents are responsible for their children. What it does mean is that parents look toward the future, wanting egalitarian relationships for their child's adult life. Most important, parental authority over children is given by the child willingly through respect of the parent, not force or fear.

In an opinion piece in a metropolitan newspaper, a proud mom says some spanking is useful. "I spanked my son sparingly in his early years, and he became a productive member of society. He graduated from college cum laude and is now a colonel in the Marine Corps Reserve working on a master's degree and a pilot for Delta. Just sayin.'"⁴ She and her husband were spanked, and both grew up to respect authority, one of the more prominently cited reasons for the usefulness of spanking. However, teaching kids to respect authority may not be the goal of modern parents. Contemporary parents want to teach their children how to voice their values without shutting others out, accept when they have made mistakes and be willing to right them, innovate and think independently, and cooperate with others in society rather than only respect others' authority.

When we hit our kids, we are knocking something out of them. Historically, it was believed to be the badness, the wickedness in the human child. But it may also be the spirit, the goodness, their gifts that get beaten out too. Can we stifle that special human spirit if we discipline too harshly? A reframing of the inborn nature of children as gifts to nurture and shape has replaced the idea of bad seeds to snuff out. Parents want a little bit of spirit in their kids, some spunk—it gives hope.

And so we have come full circle. One of the last parenting books to openly discuss spanking, a parenting guide from 1993 that advocated for spanking as a useful disciplinary tool, called out a special section on the danger of spanking too soon. The authors of *Parent Talk: Straight Answers to the Questions that Rattle Mom and Dad* caution, "First, you run the risk of extinguishing the child's spirit. Breaking the child's will is how you teach him to be responsible and accountable, but breaking his spirit shatters his self-image and leaves him with low self-esteem. Second, you run the risk of raising a child who will be too powerful, and he'll learn to use power just as it was used on him. What you are teaching the child is that Mommy or Daddy is bigger and more powerful, and that is really what's important in life, being powerful."[5]

Insight from a Jewish perspective on human nature, one I learned from my trove of parenting books, Wendy Mogel's *Blessings of a B Minus: Using Jewish Teaching to Raise Resilient Teenagers*, clarified this for me. In traditional Jewish teaching each child holds an aggressive impulse that can lead to selfishness, but it is also the source of "animating energy."[6] Teachings of Judaism suggest the best lived life is one in which the animating energy, or "Yetzer Hara," is balanced with self-understanding and self-control. Our job as parents isn't to stamp out our child's unique energies and impulses but to help channel them into ways that will make them and the people around them happier. A child's gift and passion need to be cared for and respected. Parental guidance and compassion, offered intentionally by parents, is considered the "seed" of human empathy. Without such a seed, adult compassion cannot grow.[7] Mogel suggests parents should fit the discipline to the child's temperament and personality, making sure it includes love, and lots of it.

Touch

Psychologist Harry Harlow's studies in the 1950s with Rhesus monkeys focused on the experience of touch, mainly through the concept of parent–infant bonding. His study paired an infant Rhesus monkey with a wire mesh "parent" that contained a food source and a wire mesh "parent" covered in a soft cloth. His discovery of the Rhesus monkey's preference for the cloth-covered parent stunned the psychological research community, who had believed that much of parent–child bonding was related to parents as a food source. Harlow's contribution to the importance of physical touch in the lives of young species spawned a new direction in social and psychological research. Touch is a powerful way of understanding and perceiving one's body and one's meaning to and distinction from others. As far back as 1950, we knew that touch affects a person's understanding of their body.[8] The early years of life are especially prone to touch as the infant is completely cared for. While caring for small children, parents are touching them about 50% of the time.[9] In infancy, parents hold babies frequently, make sounds like cooing, and use touch and facial expressions to soothe an irritated child. These body experiences are the primary means of how one learns to relate to others.

"Under normal conditions, parents are the most significant people in the development of the child's body image, for the interaction with parents imparts an indelible impression on the child."[10] When these interactions are positive, the child learns they are loved and cared for and is able to extend love and care to others. Touch is instrumental to our human development. From the book, *Touch: The Foundation of Experience*:

> Touch is a fundamental, possibly necessary component of the development of the earliest social attachment bonds. Attachment bonds are central to the normal development and integrative functioning of the high primates, especially man. Their presence is associated with pleasurable states, and good physical health. Their absence, or disruption, is associated with dysphoria, and increased risk of impaired health; their inappropriate disruption may constitute a major psychobiological insult to the organism.[11]

Touch communicates and has long-lasting effects on a child's development.[12] Parent touch provides a regulating function, a communication tool; even being in proximity to the child, our facial expressions, posture, tone of voice, and eye contact communicate to our child. Touch is rarely experienced in a singular sense but is combined with emotion, language, and visuals that make touch a complex human experience to understand. Parents are emotional coaches to their children, demonstrating how to express themselves in interactions.[13] Often, soothing techniques fade as the child ages, replaced by directions and discipline, possibly quicker than the child needs. Parents appropriately expect more independence, but leaping from soothing to swatting fails to match the pace of human development. The most positive communication patterns between parent and child include relaxed movements and soft facial expressions, close proximity as well as attentiveness. As children age, positive touch from parents includes patting, stroking, holding hands, hugging, and physically guiding the child in a gentle way.[14] When parents do this, the child reciprocates this same pattern in return. It is a connection.

All touch between parent and child builds a form of attachment, but not all kinds of touch are healthy. Physical punishments such as slapping and hitting are messages, a form of communication shared by touch.[15] When hitting is used as a common form of touch, it is learned as a way in which family problems are handled and as the way love and power are demonstrated.[16] Any kind of touch, even negative ones, have rewards. Spanking feels like it brings the parent and child together because the physical closeness of how their bodies interact beyond the buttocks and the hand sends messages.[17] There is an emotional buildup before the spanking, escalating attention to each other.

It culminates in the parent and child coming close together, face to face and then face to rump. There is a strong emotional connection at this time, even if it is deeply stressful. The parent may be experiencing anger and the child fear, but they are sharing a heightened emotional experience.[18] This creates a form of connection too, a much more stressful one, but it is a connection. If hitting involves the only, or most intense forms of, emotional interaction between parent and child, that connection powerfully shapes children's understanding of human touch and connection. Fear of spanking increases the child's desire to connect to their parents for any kind of comfort and sense of safety they can get.[19] Moreover, the secrecy of the spanking creates a kind of solidarity between parent and child. A scary but intimate secret. These misguided feelings of connection during and after a spanking confuse parents into believing they have created a credible and teachable experience for their child.

Trauma

While we know healthy touch is an indisputable need for the growing infant and child, the impact of touch that causes pain is understood through the study of maltreatment and trauma. The definition we must grapple with is that inside family homes many people do not view spanking as real hitting, nor would they categorize it as trauma or maltreatment. If they did, far fewer people would participate. Nonetheless, spanking is hitting, and it may occur daily or twice a year, but over the course of our life being hit adds up. In describing the psychological impact of being physically punished, Robert Greven states, "Our minds and bodies absorb the blows and pain in childhood and react to them in a multitude of ways for the remainder of our lives, forming a substratum of early experience that continues to be manifested in an astonishing variety of forms in our adult psyches."[20]

Our psyche remembers the hitting, but our body shares in the memories too. "The body is where we live. It's where we fear, hope and react. It's where we constrict and relax. And what the body most cares about are safety and survival. When something happens to the body that is too much, too fast, or too soon, it overwhelms the body and can create trauma."[21] Resmaa Menakem is a social worker and somatic therapist who outlined this process in his book, *My Grandmother's Hands: Racialized Trauma and the Pathways to Mending Our Hearts and Bodies*. Menakem notes that lived experiences form a body memory that each of us carries with us. We are often unaware of this carrying of memory in our body, long after the trauma has ended. These bodily memories are often integrated into a person's life, becoming part of their personal narrative, sometimes even being labeled as a personality defect. The spirit of even small, harsh bodily messages is retained and shapes family dynamics. Once that pattern is established, and if it is re-established, it gets harder to shift from. *That child is naughty. That child is always talking back. That parent loses his cool.* Our empathy is lost, and our positive stories about the child or parent are gone, and the negative perspective becomes so deeply entrenched that the child grows up and becomes who they were described to be. This shapes the continued life of the child and parent and becomes identified as personality, family dynamics, even culture.[22]

Trauma can spread between family members too, such as when unchecked rage is thrown at others as a mechanism to deal with one's own pain, often unexpectedly. If behaviors like hitting and spanking become normalized and accepted in the family, they become solidified into family dynamics, creating a source of continuous traumatic experiences.[23] While our body remembers, our intellect justifies and judges. *I am bad and deserved it. My mother is so erratic. My parents never listen.* Our physical bodies and our emotional and cognitive selves are connected. The ability to be calm and secure begins in the body, not in the mind. A parent and child can both feel unsafe in a spanking event, fearful that the parent may go too far, that physical injury will occur, and that the shared bond of love will begin to disintegrate. Even fear that the spanking won't work. Frequency adds up in our memories too. The more frequently we recall childhood spankings as an adult, the more likely we are to recall our childhood as abusive.[24]

Spanking, combined with enormous love from parent to child, intertwines unhealthy ways of learning about love as submission to authority, combined with fear and rejection. The experience of anxiety and fear, the hand of the parent striking the butt of the child, and the pain from someone a child loves so dearly, along with the command that the child not resist, can lead to warped expectations of loving relationships.[25] Our "inner child" stays with us as we transform into adulthood, shaping our relationships. Sometimes our inner child needs to be reckoned with, even parented by one's self. In *Your Inner Child of the Past*, author Hugh Missildine states: "[Y]our childhood and the child you once were are not something wholly behind you, long ago and far away. Your childhood, in an actual, literal sense, exists within you now. It affects everything you do, everything you feel."[26] Memories of childhood can be vague or clear, but we have them for a reason.[27] For the memories to stick, they must have a strong impact on us emotionally, visually, or physically. They can even be the source of how we feel right now: anxious, relaxed, hurt, happy—evoking the same feelings from long ago.

Frequency, duration, location, sensation, intensity, and accumulation of spankings matter. So does the look in a parent's eyes, the shape of their mouth, their breathing and tone of voice. Our brains register these bodily changes in the seconds that it takes to warn, grab, hit, and stomp away from a child. Parental expressions of shame, love, forgiveness, laughter, and anger are remembered by us too. Put these experiences under the scope of time, the 18 years it takes to raise a child, and meaningful differences are likely to occur. Bessel van der Kolk, in his book *The Body Keeps the Score*, reminds us that parents don't just dress, feed, and take care of a child's instrumental needs. Parents are shaping brains while interacting with their children, helping them understand reality. These interactions "form the template of how we think of ourselves and the world around us. These inner maps are remarkably stable over time."[28] They influence us for the rest of our lives.

We can create trauma, but we can create resiliencies too. Resilience can be passed on and shared with others and include memories of being loved and cared for, feelings of safety, problem-solving, and a sense of belonging. *We figured it out. My parents are proud of my efforts. I want to do better. I am forgiven and loved.* Like trauma, we carry these experiences within ourselves. When stresses in life emerge, different kinds of memories flood our cognitive and emotional systems, and hence our bodies. When we are our best selves, we have memories of kindness, making it through tough times, learning, and even thriving.[29]

Brain Development and Health

What we didn't know in generations past was information on brain development and how it sets us up for a lifetime of experiences. A child's brain is born programmed to grow and respond to the world around it. Goleman, the author of *Social Intelligence*, states, "[A] child's brain shapes itself to fit its social ecology, particularly the emotional climate fostered by the main people in her life."[30] If positive experiences are not common enough, even a seldom-experienced negative action will have a large impact.[31] Being hit, including spanking, affects brain development, impairs development of children, changes biology, and has lasting consequences.[32] We now know that the experiences we have change the expression of our biology. Highly charged spanking experiences leave their stamp on our development, including findings of slowed cognitive development.[33] Kids who are spanked have altered functioning in their brains, including reduced volumes in brain matter development.[34] Children also have non-normal and increased activation in multiple parts of the brain in response to threats or fearful facial expressions, depleting brain resources for social-cognitive processing.[35] No matter where we live in the world, or our wealth status, spanking inhibits children's social-emotional development.[36] The fear of being spanked again can produce a hypervigilance, especially if the reasons for a spanking are arbitrary or unclear. The child can't determine what behavior might bring on a spanking, causing worry, fear, and vigilance. Potential spankings can be a major source of worry for some children.[37] We don't even have to be participating in the hitting to be affected. Watching a sibling be hit or a co-parent hitting your child can cause secondary trauma.

Our brain and body synchronize with those around us. Parent–child is one of our closest human relationships, and our biological states take cues from each other. When people around us are calm or stressed, our bodies synchronize with them and share similar feelings. This synchrony occurs between parent and child across the child's development, not just in infancy.[38] Parent and infant synchronize their emotional and physical states,[39] which explains how children learn over time; as they watch others and mimic their behaviors, they mimic their emotions too.[40] Mirror neurons in our brains explain important aspects of this synchrony like empathy, imitation, and language. In some ways our mirror neurons make us vulnerable because we are so open and influenced by others' emotions, including negativity or rage.[41] Mirror neurons are automatic efforts to mirror the emotions of those in proximity, causing us to mimic each other, and this explains why emotions spread throughout a group or a family. We understand each other through these mirror neurons and synchronicity. It helps us "get" each other. It also means our emotions aren't private; other people can sense them. When interactions are satisfying and enjoyable, our brains emit oxytocin and endorphins, securing our attention to these positive feelings. The absence of shared pleasurable moments growing up are one explanation for adults who struggle to find trusting, joyful relationships.

The most potent exchanges come from the people we are closest to and spend the most time with. Our brain doesn't just drive our behavior but is shaped in a reciprocal way with others we spend time with. When people dump emotions on us, like disgust or anger, they activate those same emotions in us. We end up with a set of social experiences, some brought on by us, and others given to us.[42] Even loving looks make us feel secure and happy, and angry or distressed looks cause stress hormones to be released.

Our temperament is partly determined by biology. Our biological temperament and our experiences can inhibit or encourage angry outbursts and how quickly we recover from them.[43] Being a person who hits seems intuitively to be difficult on the adult brain and body. We only hit when we are under duress or stress. Stress is known to be unhealthy because it produces cortisol, creating long-term havoc with our health. Even years later, images, sounds, and thoughts related to traumatic touch can bring on a cascade of stress hormones inside our brains and bodies[44] Children not only feel threatened, but their bodies also exhibit high hormonal activity to that stress.[45] It is likely parents experience this too.

Epigenetics studies how experiences shape our DNA and the expression of our genetic makeup. The genes we inherit guide our biological development, but experiences, especially in childhood, change the expressions and markers on these genes, allowing for varied outcomes for all of us. Researchers call these "epigenetic signatures," and they can provide resiliency or risk. Warmth and care minimize stress and are positive ways to influence these epigenetic markers.[46] Seven out of 10 of the leading causes of death are affected by childhood trauma; it changes the shape and trajectory of our brain development, and our bodies too. Heart disease and lung cancer rates triple and cause a 20-year shortened life expectancy. Childhood trauma gets "under our skin and changes our physiology."[47]

A child's gene expression is shaped by thousands of routine daily interactions experienced over years of parenting experiences; marking individual parenting moments as important, but even more significant is the overall tone and feeling of these interactions. If our brains are shaped to expect mistrust, fear, rejection, and anxiety, our future relationships can struggle to diverge from that. But if love, trust, care, and safety are the norm, then adult relationships can follow that pattern, influencing our adult friendships and romantic relationships. In *A Natural History of Love*, Diane Ackerman states, "How we love is a matter of experience."[48]

The ACE You Never Want

Child abuse is harmful. We also know that other kinds of experiences during childhood can be adverse to kids' development. In 1998 researchers began to measure the long-term impact of specific negative experiences during childhood. In addition to child abuse, they identified having family members with mental illness, incarceration, substance abuse, and several other events as experiences of adversity that impact the long-term health and well-being of children. They named the measurement tool the Adverse Childhood Experience (ACE) questionnaire. The initial research found that adults with higher scores on the ACE demonstrated multiple risk factors for adult problems like depression, alcoholism, and drug abuse, and the leading causes of death in adulthood such as heart, liver, and lung diseases.[49] The findings were astonishing and made significant waves in the psychological research world. It was clear evidence that our childhood experiences are so powerful they influence our entire life span.

In 2017 an analysis of the ACE questionnaires included data on spanking. The findings revealed that spanking measures similarly to other forms of child abuse. Researchers realized that spanking results are so similar to abuse that they create the same outcomes as for kids who were physically abused.[50] The ACE study showed that childhood spanking increases suicide attempts, excessive drinking patterns, and street drug use in adulthood, long after the spankings have ended. Our understanding, treatment, and prevention of adult mental health impairments grow drastically when we realize spanking is a form of child abuse.[51]

This Is Gonna Hurt Me More Than You

Parenthood changes us. People may choose not to work and parent full-time or set aside hobbies they love. When we use parenting and discipline tactics that support the development of parents and who they are becoming, parents can have a transformational experience too. Parenthood forces us to make priorities. "This is gonna hurt me more than you" has been used by parents to justify hitting their child. The adage may be more true than we expected. When we hit other people, especially if we are feeling anger, our stress hormones increase, and it harms our health.[52] Hitting someone we love is a form of trauma for the parent, so much so that parents sometimes block it out. Many parents don't remember spanking their kids, and when grown children ask them to recount the events in which they spanked them, they simply cannot remember.[53]

One of the most important parental roles is to create and sustain loving family dynamics. Hitting counters this goal, making it harder to build positive family interactions. Negative feelings may persist long after the spanking is over. Parental efforts to rationalize the spanking as "necessary" or "for their own good" can feel very different to the child, who may view the spanking only in service to the parent. Most problematic, spanking makes parents' discipline worse. Parents who spank mildly are at higher risk for spanking harshly a year later.[54] For many parents, a harsh verbal message is simultaneous with the spanking. "You are so naughty!" or "I'm sick of your behavior, knock it off!" Physical punishment can involve a "double dose" of pain; the physical pain produced by the spanking and the emotional pain of the accompanying words.[55] Parents find they have less control over their child and themselves over time, the opposite of what they are aiming for. In her work on Premeditated Parenting, Dr. BraVada Garrett-Akinsanya, a psychologist, therapist, and activist for 30 years, believes that one of the best clinical tools for therapists is to empathize with parents who spank. Most parents are hurt by spanking, and they want to stop, but they may not have the tools to do so.[56]

Parents may feel overwhelmed and underskilled with a child who appears to outwit them at every turn. This can impair a parent's sense of self. But when all the blame is on the child, it stunts parental growth. In *The Mother Dance*, Harriet Lerner writes, "When I can view our shortcomings as parents with curiosity and self-love, I can do the same for my kids."[57] One mother who hit her daughter with a belt felt powerless after each event. She felt she shouldn't have to hit her to get the respect she wanted, so she quit.[58] Feelings of powerlessness are common in spankers. The last resort idea is true: Parents don't know what else to do; they trust this final effort will help change their child, and when it doesn't, they feel they have no further options.

Even a mild spanking of one's child, can trigger long-lost feelings and memories for the parent. Memories of a parent's own physical discipline and seeing themselves repeat those behaviors brings the harm of the parents' past onto their child. Spanking causes negative effects for the parent, even after the spanking.[59] Sometimes during the spanking the parent may disassociate, a kind of zoning out. After the spanking, rather than processing the trauma, they rationalize the event in an attempt to reduce feelings of shame. These triggered memories revive the emotional energy of past events, bring them forward to the current reality, and continue the negative biochemical responses in the body.[60]

Parents attempting to gain compliance through physical punishment lose out on developing their communication skills. The threshold for how much communication parents try before hitting their child varies. A parent who limits their communication efforts will prematurely conclude that the child is stubborn or naughty and that a spanking is required. They perceive the communication problem in the receiver rather than in themselves. They spank the child, reasserting the authority that allows people with power to have a voice and not others.[61] When parents utilize more verbal messages in more creative ways to their child, they are more likely to create a situation in which spanking is not needed.[62] As a bonus, parents stretch their communication skills—skills useful at home and in the rest of their lives.

The first place we practice new behaviors is often inside our family home; we then take those skills out into the world around us. This is as basic as learning to make a sandwich. But it also includes how to express conflict, or work together to get something done, and how to learn from others. Adults are still practicing these skills. Outside the home, spanking is not a skill any parent can use. Learning to channel one's emotions and skills into behaviors that promote respect, protectiveness, conflict resolution, and leadership in times of stress are some of the most complex expectations we have for adults. Managing your own emotions and helping others manage theirs are a highly respected part of emotional intelligence. These are the skills a parent could be practicing instead of spanking their kids.

Some parents defuse the potentiality for discipline and understand how to "calm the restless beasts" before a disciplinary incident occurs as a way to reduce spanking. You've seen a scenario like this before. You are with other parents at a friend's home or neighborhood playground. The parents enjoy each other's company as the kids begin to play and giggle. The parents barely need to notice. About an hour in, there is a nearly imperceptible crack in the perfection of the situation. It's hard to describe. The kids aren't frustrated yet, but you can feel the shift in the air. The parents start paying attention, though they don't need to intervene yet. The parent with the "spirited" child has to intervene first. The parents begin to pack up, give directions to their kiddos while they are still capable of following simple commands, and begin to exit. Playtime is over. Perceptive parents know when a meltdown is coming. When parents move forward with a sense of integrity, of maintaining respect and dignity for themselves and their child, they can sometimes avoid the need for discipline. When you start to prevent negative behaviors, you'll feel more capable, not less. The stress of life won't be gone, but you'll feel more resilient and capable.

If parents let the stressful event happen, they may find themselves spanking harder than expected when the stressors from a public meltdown feel overwhelming, compounding the difficulties of the situation the parent is in. "But it is not enough to say it is normal for parents to be angry with their children, just as it is normal for children to feel furious with their parents. We also must look at what our anger is doing to us,"[63] says Nancy Samalin in *Love and Anger: The Parental Dilemma*. The trials of parenting can be terrifying at times, and the consequences of doing it wrong feel severe. On the day I decided not to spank my kids I felt I had freed myself from an expectation I wasn't sure I could adequately fulfill. Removing spanking from my parenting repertoire made things easier. How does hitting someone we love shift and change the ways in which we view ourselves? If it hurts us more than it hurts them, is it still worth it? I had taken on a different level of awareness: Disciplining my kids shouldn't hurt either of us. I wanted it to transform both of us, for the better.

The Nested Circles Once Again

Under what circumstances do children in a society thrive? They thrive in societies where the success or failure of an individual child does not rest on the skills and capacities of their parents alone. "If there is any pattern to be found in the variety of families that have succeeded and failed over the course of history, it is that children do best in societies where child-rearing is considered too important to be left entirely to parents."[64]

Historically, around the world, there is an astonishing variety of healthy family forms and childrearing arrangements and patterns.[65] Misunderstanding can occur when we fail to see the behaviors of families couched in time and cohorts, varying by geography and culture, access to information, changing advice of experts, and recognition that each child receives a response from parents unique to them. Social factors outside the family do alter parenting behaviors as parents attempt to adapt to changing social expectations. Maybe spanking worked when social norms were more rigid, when there were fewer social freedoms for how a family can be.

All kinds of worldwide violence is in decline. Steven Pinker's robust story of human violence traces the slow but detectable decline, over millennia, in war and homicide and even spanking. He attributes some of this change to the rights revolution, a wave of revolutionary efforts to provide civil rights, women's rights, and children's rights. This tide of expanding human rights does not turn easily. But it turns. The downfall of spanking is likely to occur. Children represent the future of individual families, and the monetary and time investments required to raise them will steer families away from tactics that may cause barriers to their children's success. The progress worldwide in banning physical punishment of children is likely to continue its steady march. Using morality and human rights language, the hitting of children will end. There is no moral argument that can support hitting, and the right not to be hit will be recognized across the life span rather than only in adulthood. The sanctioning of hitting children will be identified as age discrimination.

Those of us who hold strong beliefs for or against spanking can often find our anchors at either end of the spectrum. The more extreme our view on spanking, the more coherent the argument because it is often anchored in another well-known belief system.[66] If you are pro-spanking, these beliefs may be anchored in respecting parental authority, being a strong and committed parent, and the rightness of certain behaviors and the wrongness of others. If you are anti-spanking, you may find your position anchored in beliefs of morality and human rights, or that behavior must be modeled to be taught. As we edge away from either polarized position, the arguments wane, and the belief systems become more dynamic and responsive to reality. The conversation about spanking needs to start in a shame-free place without fear or intimidation. People can't get real when they are worried about their parenting being evaluated. Brenee Brown said, "You can't claim to care about the welfare of children if you're shaming other parents for the choices they're making."[67] Doing so is the cause of a divide, the place where we hold staunchly to a position on spanking and lose the connection to parents who may see things a bit differently.

We are all adapting in each moment of our lives. We repeat our experiences growing up, and we change. My mother, raised by her grandmother, recalls one of her childhood warnings, hollered in German: "I'll hit you once, so hard, your teeth will fly out your rear-end!" A warning to her and her brother that a whupping was coming if they didn't change their behavior. While my mother grew up to spank her five children and threaten them with a naughty stick, it wasn't as harsh as what she had experienced a generation before. And my children, never spanked, have a different experience. My family story is likely more common than not. Over the past few hundred years, we have ended child labor, provided free education until adulthood, created laws to stop the physical abuse of children, broadened higher education and college accessibility, and extended health care benefits through parental employment to children up to age 26. The trajectory of all our lives has improved with these changes.

If we respond with flexibility, some common sense, and even a dash of humility, most of us can be parents that are good enough. Making mistakes in a few areas won't define us as dysfunctional or dangerous. Parenting is harder yet easier than what we or family experts or researchers can see. Easier because children are resilient enough to survive and even thrive under parental mistakes and harder because some forces affecting our children are too hard for parents to even penetrate or influence.[68] Hardest to influence are the factors that weigh heavily on families like poverty, racism, and illness. Parenting is a marathon not a race. It's the repetition of poor parenting that causes problems, not the one-off bad parenting moments. We will err frequently when doing something as complex and prolonged as raising human beings.[69] There are so many intervening variables in the life of a child that as long as parental efforts are caring and intentional, most things will turn out alright.

Society's acceptance of family members hitting each other has been fading over the last 150 years. Seventy-five years ago, using a switch from a tree would have been typical in a spanking, and yet it is not accepted today. The threshold for what is acceptable has lowered considerably, and it has been in children's and parent's best interest. The way forward doesn't just prevent maltreatment from occurring but also bravely embraces the promotion of healthy parenting and healthy childrearing.[70] Modern parents want to find a way of *being* a parent, a meaningful path with mutual benefits. For the modern family, the way forward recognizes the benefits to the child—and their parents.

10

Leaving Spanking Where It Belongs

Behind Us

My boy was just like me.
He'd grown up just like me.[1]

—Harry Chapin

When I first began this book, I was sure I would provide directions for spanking, such as "how-to-spank-with-some-measure-of-safety" tips. My first drafts of this book included those step-by-step directions on how to spank a child. I rationalized that spanking is common, and to think I could end spanking by writing a book seemed audacious and maybe even misplaced. If so many people spank, and spanking is the leading indicator of child abuse, I hoped to help children avoid long-lasting trauma and parents avoid the awful guilt of hurting their child.

But my years of reading and writing changed that. I set out to take this singular parental activity and break it down into smaller parts to map the terrain of what it means to hit the people we love most who are smaller and weaker than us. I didn't set out to write a book on parenting, or love, or shame, or people's rights. But that is where the analysis led me. After 10 years of reading, talking, and analyzing spanking, I cannot give directions—even in the hopes of producing safer spanking practices. I have learned too much. I am no friend to children or adults if I tell people how to hit a human being smaller than them. It cannot be justified. Like evolutionary baggage, any purpose spanking ever had is long gone—washed away with new knowledge, respect for others, and most surprisingly, love and care for human growth and development across the entire human life span. That means parents too.

Bill Moyers interviewed the author and social critic E. L. Doctorow, who stated, "When ideas go unexamined and unchallenged for a long enough time, certain things happen. They become mythological and they become very, very

Spanked. Christina L. Erickson, Oxford University Press. © Oxford University Press 2022.
DOI: 10.1093/oso/9780197518236.003.0010

powerful. They create conformity. They intimidate."[2] The idea that spanking is necessary to raise children to be responsible adults has intimidated us to conform, even when it does not make logical sense. Hitting people, especially small people who we love, has gone unchallenged long enough. Sanctifying hitting a part of the body that is covered by clothing is covert. Believing children are always wrong and parents are always right is untruthful. Hitting people smaller than us fuels feelings of shame and powerlessness. And through the nested circles, the negative reverberations are carried over into the span of our whole lives and even our communities.

Hitting our family members makes all our chances of a joyful and trouble-free life far lower. And so I end with one request. Stop hitting people smaller, weaker, and with fewer resources than you. Find another way. Your choices are nearly endless. If you are wondering, even struggling, about your skills as a parent, welcome that as a sign of thoughtful parenting. You don't have to be sure of yourself. There is no final destination in parenting; it's a lifelong journey that can help you understand more of yourself in a great unfolding of your maturity. Intentional and caring parenting is a contribution to a child, and it will contribute to your own growth. Family interactions and parenting tools either diminish or nurture that unfolding process. A parent's job is to choose the best tool they can and make those interactions ones that bring joy and kindness, love and maturity. When we do, things like resentment, anger, and trauma begin to take up less space in our lives.

New Perspectives and Tools

We know that each of us operates with perspectives that we are not fully aware of. And all humans participate in cycles of circular causality, especially inside our families. Our parenting concerns may fuel action to quell problems, but we don't have to force change. We just need to notice and then question. Is that what I want in my child or myself? If not, notice some more, and begin to see the patterns and perspectives that shape your thinking and influence your behavior. Then, notice how they influence the most important people around you. If you want to change something, do the smallest things first. Untighten your brow, smile at your child, take a deep breath, name your best quality, name your child's. Small changes can make big differences, especially in a heated, frustrated, or challenging moment.

Take these changes a step further. What are the major values you want to instill in your children? List them out. Things like respect, kindness, and the ability to problem-solve come to my mind. Keep your values close as you think about your parenting options. Teaching children better behavior isn't easy. The following questions will help you determine what is best for your child, what reflects your values, and also what is best for you.

1. **Are your expectations of your child developmentally accurate?**
   Parents become anxiety-ridden if they feel their children are behaving badly, even when their child is not developmentally able to act differently. Ask yourself, "Is my child developmentally able to behave the way I want them to?" If not, consider yourself a teacher at that moment, not a disciplinarian.

2. **Does the child's behavior go against your values at any age the behavior is displayed?**
   A child frankly stating how they feel might be rude to you at age 3, but exactly what you aspire to in a 16-year-old. This too is a teachable moment. Give the child an example of how they can express themselves, let them practice. You don't want to snuff out this behavior, you want to shape it. This is very different from stealing, which would be against your values at any age.

3. **Is the child aware of the mistake they made?**
   Make sure your child understands they did something wrong. They may not be aware of what occurred. This will require you to converse with them. If the mistake was made by more than one child, it is best to have the same discipline for all kids and let them know they are in it together. Don't single out your child when circumstances or a group mistake may have influenced their understanding of right and wrong.

4. **Think about the temperament of your child and the layered nests they live in.**
   How can you protect your child's sense of self-worth and integrity and help them understand they made a mistake? How does your child learn? What else is happening in their life? Do they experience benefits that build their resilience or risks to their self-worth? Ask yourself, do my child's nested circles have more risks or benefits?

5. **Can the discipline tool you are using grow with your child?**
   Simple talking can become complex conversations as the child ages. Are you having a heartfelt conversation? If you've never had a conversation with your child, don't assume it will feel natural to start when they become a 12-year-old. It will be even more difficult to create a normalized conversation if you haven't done so all along. Babble with your baby, speak simply to your 3-year-old, and listen with intention all through the years.

6. **Ask yourself, "Is my child aware that they are deeply loved by me?"**
Is my child suffering or struggling? What may magnify any disadvantages?
Have I made sure the discipline I use conveys love and not loathing? Have
I listened to my child?

7. **Think about you.**
Think about who you are, the person you want to be in the world. Let go of
fear for your child. Listen to your heart and mind. What discipline can you
give that will help you be a better parent? What will help you develop new
skills? Does your nested circle have more risks or benefits?

8. **Co-parenting exercise**
You may co-parent with someone who has a different view of spanking
than you. Ask them to join you in a conversation so that you can understand each other more. Take pencil and paper, and each of you write the
word "spank" in the center of a blank sheet of paper. Now, around the word,
in free form, write down all other words that come to mind about spanking.
Freely associate other terms and ideas that the word spank makes you think
of. After you have run out of ideas, you can stop and begin a conversation
about what the two of you wrote. Just listen and share and see what you
learn about your co-parent's perspective.

You can take it a step further with your kid's crayon box. Pull out red,
yellow, and green. Every word you associate with spank that feels scary
or harmful color red. Each word that seems neutral or insignificant color
yellow. Every word that you associate with love and care color green.
Compare with your parenting partner again. What can you learn about
each other's views on spanking? Where are you the same and where do
you differ? Comment on what you understand your partner's responses to
mean. Ask if you interpreted them correctly. How does it influence your
thinking now? You can take this conversation another step further. What
shared values do you want to instill in your children? List them. If you
choose to discipline differently from each other, share how you expect each
other to hold close to the values you both wish to instill.

Options

You don't have to spank a child to help them learn, to express family leadership, or
to be a good and caring parent. You can be strong and influential and teach them
without physical force. There are many options. Choose what you believe will best
fit you and your child. And let's be real, parents and kids can feel big emotions.
Parents need a few ideas in the heat of the moment that can benefit them too.[3]

- Laugh and smile a lot when your child is behaving well, give your child affection, tell them stories, and find the beauty in them.
- Avoid situations in which negative behaviors often occur. You'll both feel less stressed.
- Offer time-in when your child is behaving well, private time for the parent and child.
  - Pleasure gaze—just look at each other with love. Smile.
  - Breathe together, pretend you're blowing up a balloon.
  - Trace the hands of each other, and talk about the similarities and differences.
- Ignore mild misbehavior that is not harmful.
- Child-proof a space when possible; remove items you don't want the child to interact with.
- In downtime, give your child choices of activities you already approve of so that boredom does not lead to negative behaviors.
- Notice when your child behaves well, and tell them.
- Allow your child a chance to talk about their behaviors and feelings, especially during times they have made mistakes. Encourage them as they struggle with their limited words. Tell them you are happy to see them trying so hard to speak carefully and truthfully.
- Don't ask your child, "Why did you do that?" That question is too hard to answer and can feel accusatory. Ask your child questions that begin with how or what. Such as, "How are you feeling?" "What happened here?" "How can we make it better?" "What do you think we should do now?"
- Ask your child to participate in setting the learning experiences or consequences for their misbehavior.
- Give a time out for your child and you.[4]
- Help your child choose a way to make amends and heal. Nothing is more important than making things right again. Clean something up, pay someone back, provide care to someone they may have hurt, write an apology note.
- When there is conflict, ask yourself, how can we transform this to curiosity?[5] This will help transform the conflict into something new, often with solutions.
- Finally, consider approaches that focus on the good things your child, and you, do every day. What we pay attention to grows.

Modern life calls us to display far more complex skills than hitting when we are frustrated, want to teach, or even punish. It takes practice to learn these skills, model them, and teach them to others. Start now. We all get better at it with time. And even if the result isn't perfect. No one got hit. No shame or guilt or make up needed. No worry of injuries, no risk of trauma.

Ending the Hitting of Children

The complete ending of spanking children is a difficult goal to reach. But that can't stop adults and parents, as well as professionals like social workers, teachers, school administrators, nurses, and pediatricians, from advocating to end the acceptance of hitting children in all its forms, including the ones we have renamed and codified as acceptable, like spanking, smacking, and whupping. Rather than seeing these forms of hitting as different and acceptable, we must see them for what they are: violent acts. Hitting may be on a continuum of harshness, but it is all violence.

When we understand spanking and school corporal punishment as a form of violence and assault, the absurdity of our long-standing acceptance of it will begin to shift. In the United States, one of the easiest places to begin is our public school system. If you live in a state that allows teachers and school administrators to hit children, call up your state representative and/or senator and ask them to draft and support a bill to outlaw school corporal punishment. If beginning in your school district is more accessible, you can begin there too. Request that the superintendent support the banning of physical punishment in your school district. When you are successful in banning corporal punishment in one school, the whole district, or a whole state, let the media know. Share the story. Congratulate the people who advocated with you and let them know that more than the children will be better off—the whole community and all of the nested circles will benefit.

Ending spanking inside the family home is challenging, but not impossible. We can't leave it up to families to do on their own. Sixty-three countries have already led the way, and many more are moving in that direction. In the United States, each state law that addresses abuse of children will need to be re-written to include all forms of physical punishment as abuse. Legislation that clearly supports a child's right to live without physical punishment is indispensable. It assures a generalized and common understanding of the legal parameters that ban hitting—whether it leaves a mark or not.[6] Legislators, social workers, child advocates, and all other professionals can join in the process of rewriting state language that clearly identifies all hitting as abuse. Child protection services in every state and county in the United States will need to adapt their practices to educate and support families with positive parenting practices, informing parents that hitting children is a form of assault. Organizations and professional groups that serve families and children can make clear statements against all forms of hitting children, including spanking.

These changes should include multifaceted education and outreach to parents at pediatric visits, faith communities, schools, and childcare centers. Empowering parents to bring forth their best selves in the parenting process is an important place to begin. Parents learning to manage their emotions, for their own self-interest, will be a positive influence on their children.

If you are a professional who works with families, begin including spanking in your discussion of what child abuse is. Let families know that any hitting is abusive and that families who hit, even in legal ways, have higher chances of being involved in the child protection system. Come out with your own story of deciding not to spank your child, or even regretting that you once did. Let others know that you've decided it's not good for parents or children. Hitting our children is harming ourselves.

Modern Authority

As my children grew through the elementary years and into middle school, life didn't seem to get easier from those toddler years. Without notice, my husband and I could find ourselves on two different tracks, racing to perform at work, take care of our home, and parent our daughters, with our personal development taking a back seat. We sometimes felt more like project managers than parents. I realized that was okay when I read Sarah Susanka's *the not so big life* book, where she describes time and intention in project management. "If we are trying to accomplish a project by frenetically racing around in a vain attempt to get everything done, the results will embody that frantic energy." Parenting is a kind of project, and we can hold it with more intention and grace, imbue it with beauty, trust it is an art as much as a science. Susanka continues, "The point is to learn as much as we possibly can about ourselves, who we are now, and who we are becoming through the process of accomplishing the task at hand. As we engage in our project— our act of creation—there's an incredible kind of nutrition available in the experiencing of every moment as the results come into being." Our children are co-creators with us in this project we call our family life. There is no way for them not to be.

Modern families would do well not to overemphasize a nostalgic parental role of complete authority. That model has its weaknesses and doesn't prepare any family member for the modern world. Families have always changed and adapted.[7] The costs of raising a single child have been estimated to be more than $1 million. Parents often spend more than two decades helping children prepare for life, often while sacrificing many of their own dreams and desires. Many may see spanking as a benign nostalgic tradition. Nostalgic ideas of what was good for the previous generation, or what built grit for our grandparents, aren't always useful in modern families. It is okay to leave them where they are . . . in the past.

Coercion, force, and violence in any human relationship has limitations. Peace educator Paul K. Chappell says, "[T]he usefulness of violence is very limited, because it cannot confront root causes."[8] Spanking doesn't help anyone understand the mistakes a child made, and it layers another pain on top of the child's problem that still exists. The hitting is trickery: The result is emotional and physical discomfort, a problem still unsolved, and the beginning of long-term problems. In fear of spoiling children, parents often resorted too far in the opposite direction, causing harshness when often patience and new learning were needed. Joan Durrant, a spanking researcher and professor of community health said in a conference presentation, "Parents need to hear that it is okay to be kind to their children; it is not spoiling."[9]

Modern authority recognizes imperfections and owns up to them as a way of moving forward and building better dimensions of ourselves. Adult or child, we will all someday come to know our imperfections, see our mistakes laid clear. It is not an easy task to face at any age. Marian Wright Edelman, the respected founder and director emeriti of the Children's Defense Fund, a voice for children and families over decades, wrote a letter to her children in her book. *The Measure of Our Success.* She recognized the difficulty of parenting and the inescapable flaws we will experience as parents; as a gift, she wrote a letter to children:

> I seek your forgiveness for all the times I talked when I should have listened; got angry when I should have been patient; acted when I should have waited; feared when I should have delighted; scolded when I should have encouraged; criticized when I should have complemented; said no when I should have said yes and said yes when I should have said no. . . . Just as parents help shape children, children help shape parents, and you have helped me grow. Thank you for being so helpful and so forbearing. . . . Parents are sometimes frail and troubled, but also strong and resilient human beings—just like you—if we get the nurturing and support all humans need. Most of us try to keep growing just as you do, although we make lots of mistakes all the time. What we owe you, our children, is our best effort to be a person worth emulating and to send through our lives a message to the future we hope you will feel is worth transmitting to your children and grandchildren.

Since hitting children is so prevalent and is related to so many negative outcomes, committing ourselves to end spanking for all children will have a massive effect on society.[10] Social pressure for improved childhood learning will erode spanking, and the recognition of the financial investment adults make in their children will make the risks intolerable. And maybe most of all, parents will find ways that help them grow and develop and become the best versions of themselves, with parenting as one of the avenues for growth and development. I hope that in a generation, finding parents who spank will be difficult.

Parenthood grants us authority. Parents, by law, morality, and necessity, have authority over their children. This will not change. A parent's job is to exercise that authority for the greater good of the family. The challenge for the parent is to live into authority in ways that bring forth their best selves and those around them—especially for those who seek and want authority from them, their children. "Authority gets a bad rap for the many ways it gets abused. . . . But the fact is that authority itself is not good or bad, it is the *how* that matters . . . the most dangerous use of authority might be when it doesn't circle back around, in questioning and conversation, or in checks and balances." The best checks and balances are woven into the relationship itself, with the people who grant us the authority—our children.[11] A parent who leads their family well and exercises that authority for the greater good of the family welcomes respect, collaboration, and their own growth along with their child's.

Methods and Final Thoughts

This book started as a one-page exploratory idea that I shared with colleagues who offered ideas and feedback. I then crafted an outline of chapters that seemed important and relevant to spanking. Over several years I completed a vast and deep literature review and analysis of journal articles from scholarly and historical materials. I recovered materials from journals, newspapers, and magazines as far back as the mid-1800s. Using the words spank, whup, paddle, physical discipline, corporal punishment, harsh parenting, and obedience, I found hundreds of articles to review. I then launched into a multiyear literature review that continued to expand the original outline.

I reviewed dozens of parenting books published between 1931 and 2018 by scanning their tables of contents and their indices for the keywords spank, whup, paddle, discipline, corporal punishment, harsh parenting, and obedience. I pulled and reviewed all books I could find that included these words. I did not review this material for any type of quality, simply relevance to spanking. For those books that referenced the topic, I did not read the whole book, but I read all the content related to the key words, as well as some of the surrounding content to make sure I captured the essence of the author's intent.

I spent several days at the Social Welfare History Archives (SWHA) at the University of Minnesota Libraries, reviewing enormous amounts of information to find any nuggets of historical spanking that I could. The SWHA holds the largest collection of North American historical literature on family education, social services, philanthropic, and socially related materials. Their capable and trustworthy archivist, Linnea Anderson, reviewed my ideas and determined which boxes, of thousands of historical materials, had the best chance of including spanking. I reviewed hundreds of materials: pamphlets, meeting minutes, case notes, booklets, letters, memorabilia, and agency and institutional papers, in the hope of finding references to spanking.

Regarding the laws on corporal punishment in schools, legal language was culled from state websites in the summer of 2018. Child abuse state laws were pulled in 2019, and international laws on corporal punishment were gathered in 2021. These have the potential to change since those points in time.

Finally, I had to make some decisions about which findings could be included. The material is vast, and the challenge was to capture the most important concepts for a digestible book. I made decisions to expand some important ideas not explored before, such as privacy of the family and parental growth and maturity. I also compressed some components because they were repetitive or did not provide a novel understanding of this well-researched topic. To do so, I used my best professional judgment honed from many years in social work and as an academic researcher and professor. Where I may have left gaps or untold findings, I trust colleagues and other caring people will come forward with new analyses and ideas.

When I began this project, my children were in elementary school, and now they are in college. I have grown and changed through the process of parenting them and the writing of this book. I trust in families, and I believe there are many ways to raise children well. And the next iteration of my life will include watching my two daughters become parents if they choose to do so. I stopped myself from spanking them; my husband never had the impulse. What will my two daughters do, and what might their partners expect? Statistically, my daughters are most likely to co-parent with partners who have been spanked, and they may want to keep up that tradition. And so, I struggle a bit. Not for the grandchildren I have never met. They are hard for me to imagine. But for my daughters and the people they love. I hope they can create a family without hitting. For them.

Book Group Questions

> I don't think there are answers in life. I think there are only really good dialogues.[1]
>
> **—Habits of the Heart**

Part I

Chapter 1: Whupping, Paddling, Smacking: A Spank by Any Other Name Still Stings

1. What is your response to the Adrian Peterson case? How does it compare with your response to the McDaniel family?
2. Have you been spanked? Tell one of your spanking memories if you feel comfortable. Reflect on how it compares to others in your book group. Find similarities and differences and simply note them.
3. Recall your growing-up years. What are some of your memories related to the following?
   a. Parental affection
   b. Sibling affection
   c. Spanking on TV
   d. Spanking in books
   e. Being in trouble
   f. Disappointing your parents
4. What do you think is the current percentage of parents who spank in your social circles?
5. Have you been hit since you were spanked? How was it different? How was it the same?
6. Why do you think we culturally accept this one form of hitting?

Chapter 2: History and Mystery

1. What surprised you about the changing experiences and roles of children over the years?
2. What is your knowledge about the spanking practices in your parent's generation? Grandparents?
3. Turning points regarding views of children began to occur in the late 1800s, bringing about more empathy for children. Are there ways in which you currently see society as having little to no empathy for children? Differences in empathy based on gender, race, or wealth status?
4. How have your social identity categories, such as age, race, gender, and religion, shaped your spanking experiences? Your childhood experiences? Your current beliefs?

Chapter 3: Limits, Laws, and Little Mary Ellen

1. The American Society for the Prevention of Cruelty to Animals set the foundation for the American Society for the Prevention of Cruelty to Children. Imagine what the arguments might have been to stretch those laws from animals to children and give an example.
2. If you have pets, do you hit them? What would you do if you saw someone hitting their pet?
3. Consider the section, *The Battered Child Syndrome*. How did C. Henry Kempe's work influence parenting practices?
4. *Appendix A, Laws on Physical Child Abuse in the United States*, covers state laws on physical child abuse. What do you notice as you read the policy language?
5. Where do the most important rights reside, with the parent or the child?
6. At what point do you think spanking crosses over into abuse?

Chapter 4: Research and Revival

1. In describing the book written by Debi and Michael Pearl, the author states that support for spanking is couched in the belief that "[a]ll behaviors of a child are rooted in explanations of badness." Have you explained childhood behaviors as "badness"? Have you interpreted a certain child's behavior as rooted in being bad?

2. Compare and contrast the stories of Straus and Dobson. Discuss how their own personal experiences influenced their message and their abilities to spread their messages.

3. What research findings were most compelling to you? Who should know about these research findings? Do you think the findings are underreported compared with information on other human behaviors such as smoking, wearing seat belts, or eating fruits and vegetables?

4. Consider the *Explanations for Negative Outcomes*. Which of these explanations are meaningful in your experience?

5. Identify an experience from your childhood in which you were disciplined by your parents. What was the discipline? If you weren't spanked, would spanking have helped or hindered your learning? Did you have a conversation with your parents? Was the conversation helpful? Explain.

Part II

Chapter 5: School Paddling: The Only Legal Place Beyond the Home

1. Did you know school paddling is legal in some states? What are your thoughts on school corporal punishment?

2. Have you or someone you know been paddled in school? If so, share the story. What is your reflection of it now?

3. Look at *Appendix B: Definition of School Corporal Punishment and Legal Language*. What do you find interesting? Share why.

4. Look at *Appendix C: School Corporal Punishment Administration and Required Parental Communication*. What do you find interesting? Share why.

5. Do you have a powerful memory, positive or negative, of a moment with a teacher or principal? What did you learn from the encounter?

6. Recall a time you misbehaved in school. How were you disciplined? Was it helpful? Would paddling have been a good option for you?

7. Would you want your children to be paddled by a teacher?

Chapter 6: Spanking Around the World

1. The author suggests that spanking could be a form of evolutionary baggage. Do you agree or disagree and why?

2. The experiences of women and children are often linked. Explain why this is. How is this true? How is it changing?
3. Is the legality of spanking a form of ageism? Explain.
4. Consider the list of countries that have banned spanking in *Appendix D: Bans on Physical Punishment of Children: Year and Country*. Have you traveled to, or do you live in, one of these countries? Can you see connections/consequences to other social issues when spanking is banned?
5. Should the country you live in maintain or ban all forms of physical punishment to children, including spanking? Give a 2-minute speech on why or why not.

Part III

Chapter 7: In the Privacy of the Home

1. Be honest about your judgments on spanking. How do you evaluate spanking?
2. Think back to a time when one of your parents, or you, overreacted to a situation in your family. Did it impact you? Explain.
3. Tell a spanking story from your growing-up years. Why did you choose the words you did? Do the words evoke emotion?
4. How do you feel about your parents' efforts to parent? How did their efforts shape you? Are there efforts to forgive them for? Thank them for?
5. When do worry and anxiety take hold in your family life? Does it cause you to react differently than you wish?
6. Can you identify any cycles of circular causality in your life? Is it a healthy cycle or an unhealthy cycle? What do you want to do about it?
7. Give examples of how children are different from each other and how that can lead to different parenting styles.
8. Do you perceive children's intentions differently than adults? Do you explain one child's behaviors with a specific intention? Is it accurate? Is it helpful?

Chapter 8: In the Public Sphere

1. Do you judge parents in public? Describe some of your common thoughts about parents who are parenting in public.

2. Do you feel that being judged by others influences a person's parenting in public? Explain.

3. Think back to the naughtiest thing you ever did as a child. How did you feel? What did you need at that moment? What did you need when you got caught?

4. Did you ever misbehave in public as a child? What were your intentions? How did your parent(s) interpret your intentions?

5. Have you ever been an adult with a misbehaving child in public? Share your story and how you felt.

6. How do you respond to adults who are struggling with a difficult child in public? Be descriptive of your behaviors. What do you do? What do you think you should do?

7. Do you do things to preserve the public display of your family? What do you do? Is there meaning to these efforts? Are they helpful or hurtful?

Chapter 9: Modern Family

1. What are the main tasks of modern parenting? Does spanking fit with those tasks?

2. What are your thoughts about your peers spanking their children? Do you judge them? Is there a spanking stigma?

3. Would you like the children you know and love to grow up and spank their children? Why or why not?

4. If you have grandchildren or hope to someday, do you feel differently about them being spanked versus your children?

5. Even though we may hold onto a nostalgic notion of an ideal family, families are always changing. What would the ideal modern family be like and what kind of relationships would exist between adults and children?

6. Bessel van der Kolk and Resmaa Menakem tell us that the body has memory. Do you feel your body has memory? In your body can you feel hope? Fear? Anticipation? Love? Rejection?

7. Who taught you about your body? What were those lessons? Are there still vestiges of that learning in your life? How would you change it? What would you teach a child about their body?

8. Recall a time in which you were spanked or you gave a spanking. Now, replay the event in your mind one more time paying attention to your body. How does your body experience the event? Your heart rate? Your muscles? Your breathing? How does your mind interpret the event?

Chapter 10: Leaving Spanking Where It Belongs: Behind Us

1. Excise the word spank from your vocabulary and replace it with hit. What changes?
2. Complete the free-association exercise on the word spank described in the book. What did you learn about your ideas and conceptions of spanking?
3. Review the section on questions to consider before choosing a disciplinary method with your child. What sections stand out to you?
4. Do you take time to listen to children? Do you allow them to practice words with you and how to express them?
5. Do adults sometimes have less compassion for children? How might adult compassion for an unsure parent or teacher be helpful?
6. Identify for yourself why spanking your children would be bad for you. What skills can you expand on and practice, instead of hitting your child?

Questions for Organizations and Professionals

Organizations

1. Does the organization you work for create welcoming spaces for children? How do patrons or clients know children are welcome?
2. Do parents, attempting to complete adult activities at your organization, have safe options to occupy their children while they conduct their business?
3. Brainstorm changes your organization could make to promote the well-being of children. Consider implementing one or two of them.
4. If you want to influence the perception of spanking in the people you work with, what might be one or two strategies you could embark on?
5. If your organization is staffed by mandated reporters of child abuse, what does your policy say about that process? Does it include spanking?
6. Can your organization take a stand on spanking children? What might that look like?
7. Could your organization support the Convention on the Rights of the Child? What might that look like?
8. Read the state law on child abuse in your state. Would you recommend changes? If so, rewrite the child abuse laws in your state. What would be essential to include? How can you go about advocating for the changes?
9. Review school corporal punishment laws in your state. Does your state allow school corporal punishment? How might you strategize a change in this law?
10. Compare state laws on child abuse with national bans on physical punishment. What do you notice?
11. Review the countries that ban physical punishment and the language they have chosen to do so. What can your organization learn from this language that may inform its own stance on physical punishment?

Professions

12. Do people in your profession influence spanking? Explain. If not, could they?

13. Does your profession have a stance on spanking? If so, how has the profession communicated it?

14. If they do not have a stance, do you think they need one? What would be the main point of the stance you would suggest for your profession? Draft a few sentences for your profession.

15. Do you have time and space for meaningful conversations about supporting parents in your profession? If not, how could you create room for that conversation?

16. Read the state law on child abuse in your state. Would you recommend changes? If so, rewrite the child abuse laws in your state. What would be essential to include? How can you go about advocating for the changes?

17. Could your profession support the Convention on the Rights of the Child? What might that look like?

18. Does your state allow school corporal punishment? How might you strategize a change in this law?

19. Review the countries that ban physical punishment and the language they have chosen to do so. What can your profession learn from this language that may inform its own stance on physical punishment?

Laws on Physical Child Abuse in the United States

Table A.1 West State Regions

Alaska	Child Abuse or Neglect means: 1. Physical injury or neglect 2. Mental injury 3. Sexual abuse 4. Sexual exploitation 5. Maltreatment of a child under the age 18 by a person under circumstances that indicate that the child's health or welfare is harmed or threatened
Arizona	Abuse means any of the following: 1. Inflicting or allowing physical injury, impairment of bodily function, or disfigurement 2. Physical injury that results from permitting a child to enter or remain in any structure or vehicle in which volatile, toxic, or flammable chemicals are found, or equipment is possessed by any person for the purpose of manufacturing a dangerous drug 3. Unreasonable confinement of a child Serious Physical Injury means an injury that is diagnosed by a medical doctor and that does any one or a combination of the following: 1. Creates reasonable risk of death 2. Causes serious or permanent disfigurement 3. Causes significant physical pain 4. Causes serious impairment of health 5. Causes the loss or protracted impairment of an organ or limb 6. Is the result of sexual abuse, sexual conduct with a minor, sexual assault, molestation of a child, child sex trafficking, commercial sexual exploitation of a minor, sexual exploitation, or incest
California	A child may be considered dependent (and subject to supervision by the Department of Social Services) under the following circumstances: 1. The child has suffered, or there is a substantial risk that the child will suffer, serious physical harm inflicted nonaccidentally upon the child by the child's parent or guardian. For the purposes of this subdivision, a court may find there is a substantial risk of serious future injury based on the manner in which a less serious injury was inflicted, a history of repeated inflictions of injuries on the child or the child's siblings, or a combination of these and other actions by the parent or guardian that indicate the child is at risk of serious physical harm. 2. The child is younger than age 5 and has suffered severe physical abuse by a parent or by any person known by the parent, if the parent knew or reasonably should have known that the person was physically abusing the child. 3. The child's parent or guardian caused the death of another child through abuse or neglect.

Continued

Table A.1 *Continued*

4. The child has been subjected to an act or acts of cruelty by the parent or guardian or a member of his or her household, or the parent or guardian has failed to adequately protect the child from an act or acts of cruelty when the parent or guardian knew or reasonably should have known that the child was in danger of being subjected to an act or acts of cruelty.

For the purposes of this subdivision, Severe Physical Abuse means any of the following:

1. Any single act of abuse that causes physical trauma of sufficient severity that, if left untreated, would cause permanent physical disfigurement, permanent physical disability, or death
2. Any single act of sexual abuse that causes significant bleeding, deep bruising, or significant external or internal swelling
3. More than one act of physical abuse, each of which causes bleeding, deep bruising, significant external or internal swelling, bone fracture, or unconsciousness
4. The willful, prolonged failure to provide adequate food

In the Penal Code: As used in this article, the term Child Abuse or Neglect includes physical injury or death inflicted by other than accidental means upon a child by another person; sexual abuse, as defined in §11165.1; neglect, as defined in §11165.2; the willful harming or injuring of a child or the endangering of the person or health of a child, as defined in §11165.3; and unlawful corporal punishment or injury, as defined in §11165.4.

Exceptions: Serious Physical Harm does not include reasonable and age-appropriate spanking to the buttocks where there is no evidence of serious physical injury.

Colorado   Abuse or Child Abuse or Neglect means an act or omission that threatens the health or welfare of a child in one of the following categories:

1. Skin bruising, bleeding, malnutrition, failure to thrive, burns, fracture of any bone, subdural hematoma, soft tissue swelling, or death, and the following applies:
   a. The condition or death is not justifiably explained.
   b. The history given concerning the condition is inconsistent with the degree or type of such condition or death.
   c. The circumstances indicate that the condition may not be the result of an accidental occurrence.
2. A controlled substance is manufactured in the presence of a child, on the premises where a child is found, or where a child resides
3. A child tests positive at birth for either a schedule I or schedule II controlled substance, unless the child tests positive for a schedule II controlled substance as a result of the mother's lawful intake of such substance as prescribed
4. A child is subjected to human trafficking of a minor for sexual servitude, as described in §18-3-504

Exceptions: Those investigating cases of child abuse shall take into account child-rearing practices of the culture in which the child participates, including the work-related practices of agricultural communities. The reasonable exercise of parental discipline is not considered abuse.

Table A.1 *Continued*

Hawaii	Child Abuse or Neglect means acts or omissions that have resulted in the physical health or welfare of the child who is under age 18 to be harmed or to be subject to a reasonably foreseeable, substantial risk of being harmed. The acts or omissions are indicated for the purposes of reports by circumstances that include, but are not limited to, the following:

1. When the child exhibits evidence of any of the following injuries, and such injury is not justifiably explained, or when the history given concerning such condition or death is inconsistent with the degree or type of such condition or death, or circumstances indicate that such condition or death may not be the product of an accidental occurrence:
    a. Substantial or multiple skin bruising or other internal bleeding
    b. An injury to skin causing substantial bleeding
    c. Malnutrition or failure to thrive
    d. Burns or poisoning
    e. Fracture of any bone
    f. Subdural hematoma or soft tissue swelling
    g. Extreme pain or mental distress
    h. Gross degradation
    i. Death
2. When the child is provided with dangerous, harmful, or detrimental drugs, provided that this paragraph shall not apply when such drugs are provided to the child pursuant to the direction or prescription of a practitioner
3. When the child has been the victim of labor trafficking under chapter 707

Idaho	Abused means any case in which a child has been the victim of conduct or omission resulting in skin bruising, bleeding, malnutrition, burns, fracture of any bone, subdural hematoma, soft tissue swelling, failure to thrive, or death, and such condition or death is not justifiably explained; the history given concerning such condition or death is inconsistent with the degree or type of such condition or death; or the circumstances indicate that such condition or death may not be the product of an accidental occurrence.
Montana	Physical abuse means an intentional act, omission, or gross negligence resulting in substantial skin bruising, internal bleeding, substantial injury to skin, subdural hematoma, burns, bone fractures, extreme pain, permanent or temporary disfigurement, impairment of any bodily organ or function, or death.

Child Abuse or Neglect means any of the following:
1. Actual physical or psychological harm to a child
2. Substantial risk of physical or psychological harm to a child
3. Abandonment

The term includes the following:
1. Actual physical or psychological harm to a child, or substantial risk of physical or psychological harm to a child, by the acts or omissions of a person responsible for the child's welfare
2. Exposing a child to the criminal distribution of dangerous drugs, the criminal production or manufacture of dangerous drugs, or the operation of an unlawful clandestine laboratory

Physical or Psychological Harm to a child means the harm that occurs whenever the parent or other person responsible for the child's welfare inflicts or allows to be inflicted upon the child physical abuse, physical neglect, or psychological abuse or neglect.

Continued

Table A.1 *Continued*

Nevada	Abuse or Neglect of a child means physical or mental injury of a nonaccidental nature, sexual abuse or sexual exploitation, or negligent treatment or maltreatment of a child caused or allowed by a person responsible for his or her welfare under circumstances that indicate that the child's health or welfare is harmed or threatened with harm. Physical Injury includes, without limitation, the following: 1. A sprain or dislocation 2. Damage to cartilage 3. A fracture of a bone or the skull 4. An intracranial hemorrhage or injury to another internal organ 5. A burn or scalding 6. A cut, laceration, puncture, or bite 7. Permanent or temporary disfigurement or loss or impairment of a part or organ of the body Excessive corporal punishment may result in physical or mental injury constituting abuse or neglect of a child.
New Mexico	Abused Child means a child to whom any of the following apply: 1. Who has suffered or is at risk of suffering serious harm because of the action or inaction of the child's parent, guardian, or custodian 2. Who has suffered physical abuse inflicted or caused by the child's parent, guardian, or custodian 3. Whose parent, guardian, or custodian has knowingly, intentionally, or negligently placed the child in a situation that may endanger the child's life or health 4. Whose parent, guardian, or custodian has knowingly or intentionally tortured, cruelly confined, or cruelly punished the child Physical Abuse includes any case in which the child exhibits evidence of skin bruising, bleeding, malnutrition, failure to thrive, burns, fracture of any bone, subdural hematoma, soft tissue swelling, or death, and any of the following apply: 1. There is no justifiable explanation for the condition or death. 2. The explanation given for the condition is inconsistent with the degree or nature of the condition. 3. The explanation given for the death is at variance with the nature of the death. 4. Circumstances indicate that the condition or death may not be the product of an accidental occurrence. Great Bodily Harm means an injury to a person that creates a high probability of death, that causes serious disfigurement, or that results in permanent or protracted loss or impairment of the function of a member or organ of the body.
Oregon	Abuse means any of the following: 1. An assault of a child and physical injury to a child that has been caused by other than accidental means, including injury that appears to be inconsistent with the explanation given of the injury 2. Threatened harm to a child that means subjecting a child to a substantial risk of harm to the child's health or welfare 3. Buying or selling a person under age 18, as described in §163.537 4. Permitting a person under age 18 to enter or remain in or upon premises where methamphetamine is being manufactured 5. Unlawful exposure to a controlled substance or to the unlawful manufacturing of a cannabinoid extract that subjects a child to a substantial risk of harm to his or her health or safety *Exceptions*: Abuse does not include reasonable exercise of parental discipline

Table A.1 *Continued*

Utah	Abuse means any of the following: 1. Nonaccidental harm of a child 2. Threatened harm of a child 3. Sexual exploitation 4. Sexual abuse 5. Human trafficking of a child in violation of §76-5-308.5 6. That a child's natural parent: 　a. Intentionally, knowingly, or recklessly causes the death of another parent of the child 　b. Is identified by a law enforcement agency as the primary suspect in an investigation for intentionally, knowingly, or recklessly causing the death of another parent of the child 　c. Is being prosecuted for or has been convicted of intentionally, knowingly, or recklessly causing the death of another parent of the child Abused Child means a child who has been subjected to abuse. Harm means any of the following: 1. Physical or developmental injury or damage 2. Sexual abuse or sexual exploitation Physical Abuse means abuse that results in physical injury or damage to a child. Severe Abuse means abuse that causes or threatens to cause serious harm to a child. *Exceptions*: The term Abuse does not include the following: 1. Reasonable discipline or management of a child, including withholding privileges 2. The use of reasonable and necessary physical restraint or force on a child in self-defense, in defense of others, to protect the child, or to remove a weapon in the possession of a child in self-defense or defense of others
Washington	Abuse or Neglect means the injury of a child by any person under circumstances that cause harm to the child's health, welfare, or safety or the negligent treatment or maltreatment of a child by a person responsible for or providing care to the child. An abused child is a child who has been subjected to child abuse or neglect. Severe Abuse means any of the following: 1. Any single act of abuse that causes physical trauma of sufficient severity that, if left untreated, could cause death 2. Any single act of sexual abuse that causes significant bleeding, deep bruising, or significant external or internal swelling 3. More than one act of physical abuse, each of which causes bleeding, deep bruising, significant external or internal swelling, bone fracture, or unconsciousness Any use of force on a child by any other person is unlawful unless it is reasonable and moderate and is authorized in advance by the child's parent or guardian for purposes of restraining or correcting the child. The following actions are presumed unreasonable when used to correct or restrain a child: 1. Throwing, kicking, burning, or cutting a child 2. Striking a child with a closed fist 3. Shaking a child younger than age 3 4. Interfering with a child's breathing 5. Threatening a child with a deadly weapon 6. Doing any other act that is likely to cause and that does cause bodily harm greater than transient pain or minor temporary marks

Continued

Table A.1 *Continued*

	The age, size, and condition of the child and the location of the injury shall be considered when determining whether the bodily harm is reasonable or moderate. This list is illustrative of unreasonable actions and is not intended to be exclusive.
	Exceptions: This chapter shall not be construed to authorize interference with child-raising practices, including reasonable parental discipline, that are not injurious to a child's health, welfare, and safety.
	Nothing in this chapter may be used to prohibit the reasonable use of corporal punishment as a means of discipline.
	The physical discipline of a child is not unlawful when it is reasonable and moderate and is inflicted by a parent, teacher, or guardian for purposes of restraining or correcting the child.
Wyoming	Abuse means inflicting or causing physical injury, harm, or imminent danger to the physical health or welfare of a child other than by accidental means, including excessive or unreasonable corporal punishment.
	Physical Injury means any harm to a child, including, but not limited to, disfigurement, impairment of any bodily organ, skin bruising if greater in magnitude than minor bruising associated with reasonable corporal punishment, bleeding, burns, fracture of any bone, subdural hematoma, or substantial malnutrition.

Table A.2 Midwest

Illinois	Abused Child means a child whose parent, immediate family member, any person responsible for the child's welfare, any individual residing in the same home as the child, or a paramour of the child's parent does any of the following:
	1. Inflicts, causes or allows to be inflicted, or creates a substantial risk of physical injury by other than accidental means that causes death, disfigurement, impairment of physical or emotional health, or loss or impairment of any bodily function
	2. Commits or allows to be committed an act or acts of torture upon the child
	3. Inflicts excessive corporal punishment
	4. Commits or allows to be committed the offense of female genital mutilation
	5. Causes a controlled substance to be sold, transferred, distributed, or given to the child under age 18, in violation of the Illinois Controlled Substances Act or Methamphetamine Control and Community Protection Act
	6. Commits or allows to be committed the offense of involuntary servitude, involuntary sexual servitude of a minor, or trafficking in persons, as defined in chapter 720, §5/10-9, against the child
Indiana	A child is a child in need of services if, before the child becomes age 18, the child's physical or mental health is seriously endangered due to injury by the act or omission of the child's parent, guardian, or custodian. Evidence that the illegal manufacture of a drug or controlled substance is occurring on the property where a child resides creates a rebuttable presumption that the child's physical or mental health is seriously endangered.
	Exceptions: This chapter does not limit either of the following:
	1. The right of the parent to use reasonable corporal punishment to discipline the child
	2. The lawful practice or teaching of religious beliefs

Table A.2 *Continued*

Iowa	Child Abuse or Abuse means any nonaccidental physical injury, or injury that is inconsistent with the history given of it, suffered by a child as the result of acts or omissions of a person responsible for the care of the child.
Kansas	Physical, Mental, or Emotional Abuse means the infliction of physical, mental, or emotional harm, or the causing of a deterioration of a child, and may include, but shall not be limited to, maltreatment or exploiting a child to the extent that the child's health or emotional well-being is endangered.
	Harm means physical or psychological injury or damage.
Michigan	Child Abuse means harm or threatened harm to a child's health or welfare that occurs through nonaccidental physical or mental injury, sexual abuse, sexual exploitation, or maltreatment by a parent, a legal guardian, or any other person responsible for the child's health or welfare or by a teacher, a teacher's aide, or a member of the clergy.
	Severe Physical Injury means an injury to the child that requires medical treatment or hospitalization and that seriously impairs the child's health or physical well-being.
Minnesota	Physical Abuse means any physical injury, mental injury, or threatened injury inflicted by a person responsible for the child's care on a child by other than accidental means; physical or mental injury that cannot reasonably be explained by the child's history of injuries; or any aversive and deprivation procedures or regulated interventions that have not been authorized by law.

Minnesota (continued):

Physical Abuse includes, but is not limited to, any of the following acts:

1. Throwing, kicking, burning, biting, or cutting a child
2. Striking a child with a closed fist
3. Shaking a child under age 3
4. Striking or other actions that result in any nonaccidental injury to a child under 18 months
5. Unreasonable interference with a child's breathing
6. Threatening a child with a weapon
7. Striking a child under age 1 on the face or head
8. Striking a child who is at least age 1 but under age 4 on the face or head, which results in an injury
9. Purposely giving a child poison, alcohol, or dangerous, harmful, or controlled substances that were not prescribed for the child by a practitioner, in order to control or punish the child; giving the child substances that substantially affect the child's behavior, motor coordination, or judgment or that result in sickness or internal injury; or subjecting the child to medical procedures that would be unnecessary if the child were not exposed to the substances
10. Unreasonable physical confinement or restraint not permitted by law, including, but not limited to, tying, caging, or chaining
11. In a school facility or school zone, an act by a person responsible for the child's care that is a violation under §121A.58 (prohibiting corporal punishment)

Substantial child endangerment means a person responsible for a child's care, by act or omission, commits or attempts to commit an act against a child under their care that constitutes any of the following:

1. Egregious harm, as defined in §260C.007, subd. 14
2. Murder in the first, second, or third degree or manslaughter in the first or second degree
3. Assault in the first, second, or third degree

Continued

Table A.2 *Continued*

> 4. Malicious punishment or neglect or endangerment of a child
> 5. Parental behavior, status, or condition that mandates that the county attorney file a termination of parental rights petition under §260C.503, subd. 2

Exceptions: Abuse does not include reasonable and moderate physical discipline of a child administered by a parent or legal guardian that does not result in an injury. Abuse does not include the use of reasonable force by a teacher, principal, or school employee, as allowed by §121A.582.

Missouri	Abuse means any physical injury inflicted on a child by other than accidental means by those responsible for the child's care, custody, and control. *Exceptions*: Discipline, including spanking, administered in a reasonable manner, shall not be considered abuse.
Nebraska	Child Abuse or Neglect means knowingly, intentionally, or negligently causing, or permitting a minor child to be placed in a situation that endangers his or her life or physical health, or causes or permits a child to be cruelly confined or cruelly punished.
North Dakota	Abused Child means an individual younger than age 18 who is suffering from abuse, as defined in §14-09-22(1), caused by a person responsible for the child's welfare. A child is abused when a parent, adult family or household member, guardian, or other custodian of any child willfully inflicts or allows to be inflicted upon the child mental injury or bodily injury, substantial bodily injury, or serious bodily injury, as defined by §12.1-01-04. A child is abused when a person who provides care, supervision, education, or guidance for a child unaccompanied by the child's parent, adult family or household member, guardian, or custodian in exchange for money, goods, or other services and while providing such services commits an offense under this section. Deprived Child means a child who is a victim of human trafficking, as defined in title 12.1.
Ohio	Abused Child includes any child to whom any of the following apply: 1. Is endangered, as defined §2919.22 2. Exhibits evidence of any physical or mental injury or death, inflicted by other than accidental means, that is inconsistent with the history given of it 3. Suffers physical or mental injury that harms or threatens to harm the child's health or welfare because of the acts of his or her parent, guardian, or custodian 4. Is subjected to out-of-home-care child abuse Endangering Children includes any of the following acts committed against a child under age 18 or a mentally or physically handicapped child under age 21: 1. Abuse, torture, or cruel abuse 2. Corporal punishment, other physical disciplinary measure, or physical restraint in a cruel manner or for a prolonged period that creates a substantial risk of serious physical harm to the child 3. Repeated and unwarranted disciplinary measures that, if continued, create a substantial risk of serious impairment of the child's mental health or development 4. Allowing the child to be on the same parcel of real property and within 100 feet of, or, in the case of more than one housing unit on the same parcel of real property, in the same housing unit and within 100 feet of, the illegal manufacture of drugs, cultivation of marijuana, or possession of chemicals for the illegal manufacture when the person knows that the act is occurring, whether or not any person is prosecuted for or convicted of the violation *Exceptions*: A child exhibiting evidence of corporal punishment or other physical disciplinary measure by a parent is not an abused child if the measure is not prohibited under §2919.22 (that prohibits cruel or excessive means of discipline.

Table A.2 *Continued*

South Dakota	Abused or Neglected Child means a child to whom the following applies:
	1. Whose parent, guardian, or custodian has subjected the child to mistreatment or abuse
	2. Who was subject to prenatal exposure to abusive use of alcohol, marijuana, any controlled drug, or a substance not lawfully prescribed by a practitioner
Wisconsin	Abuse means any of the following:
	1. Physical injury inflicted on a child by other than accidental means
	2. When used in referring to an unborn child, serious physical harm inflicted on the unborn child and the risk of serious physical harm to the child when born caused by a habitual lack of self-control of the expectant mother of the unborn child in the use of alcoholic beverages, controlled substances, or controlled substance analogs, exhibited to a severe degree
	3. Manufacturing methamphetamine in violation of §961.41(1)(e) under any of the following circumstances:
	a. With a child physically present during the manufacture
	b. In a child's home, on the premises of a child's home, or in a motor vehicle located on the premises of a child's home
	c. Under any circumstances in which a reasonable person should have known that the manufacture would be seen, smelled, or heard by a child
	Physical Injury includes, but is not limited to, lacerations, fractured bones, burns, internal injuries, severe or frequent bruising, or great bodily harm.
	Incident of Death or Serious Injury means an incident in which a child has died or has been placed in serious or critical condition, as determined by a physician, as a result of any suspected abuse or neglect that has been reported or in which a child who has been placed outside the home by a court order is suspected to have committed suicide.
	Incident of Egregious Abuse or Neglect means an incident of suspected abuse or neglect that has been reported under this section, other than an incident of death or serious injury, involving significant violence, torture, multiple victims, the use of inappropriate or cruel restraints, exposure of a child to a dangerous situation, or other similar, aggravated circumstances.

Table A.3 Northeast

Connecticut	The term Abused means that a child:
	1. Has been inflicted with physical injury or injuries by other than accidental means
	2. Has injuries that are inconsistent with the history given of them
	3. Is in a condition that is the result of maltreatment that includes, but is not limited to, malnutrition, sexual molestation or exploitation, deprivation of necessities, emotional maltreatment, or cruel punishment
Maine	Abuse or Neglect means a threat to a child's health or welfare by physical, mental, or emotional injury or impairment; sexual abuse or exploitation; deprivation of essential needs; lack of protection; or failure to ensure compliance with school attendance requirements under title 20-A, §3272(2)(B), or §5051-A(1)(C), by a person responsible for the child.
	Jeopardy to Health or Welfare or Jeopardy means serious abuse or neglect, as evidenced by serious harm or threat of serious harm.
	Serious harm means serious injury.
	Serious injury means serious physical injury or impairment.

Continued

Table A.3 *Continued*

Massachusetts	Abuse means the nonaccidental commission of any act by a caregiver upon a child under age 18 that causes or creates a substantial risk of physical or emotional injury, or constitutes a sexual offense under the laws of the Commonwealth, or any sexual contact between a caregiver and a child under the care of that individual.

Physical Injury means any of the following:
1. Death
2. Fracture of a bone, a subdural hematoma, burns, impairment of any organ, and any other such nontrivial injury
3. Soft tissue swelling or skin bruising depending upon such factors as the child's age, circumstances under which the injury occurred, and the number and location of bruises
4. Addiction to a drug at birth
5. Failure to thrive

New Hampshire   Abused Child means any child who has been subjected to any of the following:
1. Sexual abuse
2. Intentional physical injury
3. Physical injury by other than accidental means
4. Human trafficking by any person
5. Female genital mutilation

New Jersey   Abused Child or Abused or Neglected Child means a child under age 18 whose parent, guardian, or other person having custody and control does any of the following:
1. Inflicts or allows to be inflicted upon such child physical injury by other than accidental means that causes or creates a substantial risk of death, serious or protracted disfigurement, protracted impairment of physical or emotional health, or protracted loss or impairment of the function of any bodily organ
2. Creates or allows to be created a substantial or ongoing risk of physical injury to such child by other than accidental means that would be likely to cause death or serious or protracted disfigurement or protracted loss or impairment of the function of any bodily organ
3. Inflicts unreasonably or allows to be inflicted harm or substantial risk thereof, including the infliction of excessive corporal punishment or by any other acts of a similarly serious nature requiring the aid of the court
4. Uses excessive physical restraint upon the child under circumstances that do not indicate that the child's behavior is harmful to himself or herself, others, or property

New York   Abused Child means a child younger than age 18 whose parent or other person legally responsible for his or her care does any of the following:
1. Inflicts or allows to be inflicted upon such child physical injury by other than accidental means that causes or creates a substantial risk of death, serious or protracted disfigurement, protracted impairment of physical or emotional health, or protracted loss or impairment of the function of any bodily organ
2. Creates or allows to be created a substantial risk of physical injury to such child by other than accidental means that would be likely to cause death, serious or protracted disfigurement, protracted impairment of physical or emotional health, or protracted loss or impairment of the function of any bodily organ

Table A.3 *Continued*

Pennsylvania	The term Child Abuse shall mean intentionally, knowingly, or recklessly doing any of the following:

The term Child Abuse shall mean intentionally, knowingly, or recklessly doing any of the following:

1. Causing bodily injury to a child through any recent act or failure to act
2. Fabricating, feigning, or intentionally exaggerating or inducing a medical symptom or disease that results in a potentially harmful medical evaluation or treatment to the child through any recent act
3. Causing sexual abuse or exploitation of a child through any act or failure to act
4. Creating a reasonable likelihood of bodily injury to a child through any recent act or failure to act
5. Creating a likelihood of sexual abuse or exploitation of a child through any recent act or failure to act
6. Causing serious physical neglect of a child
7. Engaging in any of the following recent acts:
    a. Kicking, biting, throwing, burning, stabbing, or cutting a child in a manner that endangers the child
    b. Unreasonably restraining or confining a child, based on consideration of the method, location, or the duration of the restraint or confinement
    c. Forcefully shaking a child younger than age 1
    d. Forcefully slapping or otherwise striking a child younger than age 1
    e. Interfering with the breathing of a child
    f. Causing a child to be present at a location while a violation of 18 Pa.C.S. §7508.2 (relating to operation of methamphetamine laboratory) is occurring, provided that the violation is being investigated by law enforcement
    g. Leaving a child unsupervised with an individual, other than the child's parent, who the actor knows or reasonably should have known:
        i. Is required to register as a tier II or tier III sexual offender, when the victim of the sexual offense was younger than age 18 when the crime was committed
        ii. Has been determined to be a sexually violent predator
        iii. Has been determined to be a sexually violent delinquent child
    h. Causing the death of the child through any act or failure to act
    i. Engaging a child in a severe form of trafficking in persons or sex trafficking, as those terms are defined under Federal law 22 U.S.C. §7102

Exceptions: The use of reasonable force on or against a child by the child's own parent or person responsible for the child's welfare shall not be considered child abuse if any of the following conditions apply:

1. The use of reasonable force constitutes incidental, minor, or reasonable physical contact with the child that is designed to maintain order and control.
2. The use of reasonable force is necessary:
    a. To quell a disturbance or remove the child from the scene of a disturbance that threatens physical injury to persons or damage to property
    b. To prevent the child from self-inflicted physical harm
    c. For self-defense or the defense of another individual
    d. To obtain possession of weapons, dangerous objects, or controlled substances or paraphernalia that are on or within the control of the child

Continued

Table A.3 *Continued*

Rhode Island	Abused and/or Neglected Child means a child whose physical or mental health or welfare is harmed or threatened with harm when his or her parent or other person responsible for his or her welfare does any of the following:

1. Inflicts or allows to be inflicted upon the child physical or mental injury, including excessive corporal punishment
2. Creates or allows to be created a substantial risk of physical or mental injury to the child, including excessive corporal punishment

Shaken baby syndrome means a form of abusive head trauma characterized by a constellation of symptoms caused by other than accidental traumatic injury resulting from the violent shaking and/or impact upon an infant or young child's head.

Vermont	Abused or Neglected Child means a child whose physical health, psychological growth and development, or welfare is harmed or is at substantial risk of harm by the acts or omissions of his or her parent or other person responsible for the child's welfare. An "abused or neglected child" also means a child who has died as a result of abuse or neglect.

Harm can occur by physical injury.

Physical Injury means death, permanent or temporary disfigurement, or impairment of any bodily organ or function by other than accidental means.

Serious Physical Injury means, by other than accidental means, any of the following:

1. Physical injury that creates any of the following:
   a. A substantial risk of death
   b. A substantial loss or impairment of the function of any bodily member or organ
   c. A substantial impairment of health
   d. Substantial disfigurement

2. Strangulation by intentionally impeding normal breathing or circulation of the blood by applying pressure on the throat or neck or by blocking the nose or mouth of another person.

Risk of Harm means a significant danger that a child will suffer serious harm by other than accidental means, which harm would be likely to cause physical injury as the result of a single, egregious act that has caused the child to be at significant risk of serious physical injury.

Table A.4 The South

Alabama	Abuse means harm or threatening harm to the health or welfare of a child through any of the following: 1. Nonaccidental physical injury 2. Sexual abuse or attempted sexual abuse 3. Sexual exploitation or attempted sexual exploitation
Delaware	Abuse or Abused Child means that a person has care, custody, or control of a child and causes or inflicts any of the following: 1. Physical injury through unjustified force 2. Emotional abuse 3. Torture 4. Exploitation 5. Maltreatment or mistreatment Mistreatment or Maltreatment are behaviors that inflict unnecessary or unjustifiable pain or suffering on a child without causing physical injury. Behaviors included will consist of actions and omissions, ones that are intentional, and ones that are unintentional. The term "abuse" means causing any physical injury to a child through unjustified force, torture, negligent treatment, sexual abuse, exploitation, maltreatment, mistreatment, or any means other than accident. Physical injury to a child means any impairment of physical condition or pain. Serious Physical Injury means physical injury that creates a risk of death; causes disfigurement, impairment of health, or loss or impairment of the function of any bodily organ or limb; or causes the unlawful termination of a pregnancy without the consent of the pregnant female.
District of Columbia	Abused, when used in reference to a child, means any of the following: 1. Infliction of physical or mental injury 2. Sexual abuse or exploitation 3. Negligent treatment or maltreatment *Exceptions*: The term Abused does not include parental discipline, as long as the discipline is reasonable in manner and moderate in degree and otherwise does not constitute cruelty. The term Discipline does not include any of the following: 1. Burning, biting, or cutting a child 2. Striking a child with a closed fist 3. Inflicting injury to a child by shaking, kicking, or throwing the child 4. Nonaccidental injury to a child younger than 18 months 5. Interfering with a child's breathing 6. Threatening a child with a dangerous weapon or using such a weapon on a child. The above list is illustrative of unacceptable discipline and is not intended to be exclusive or exhaustive.
Florida	Abuse means any willful act or threatened act that results in any physical, mental, or sexual abuse, injury, or harm that causes or is likely to cause a child's physical, mental, or emotional health to be significantly impaired. Abuse of a Child includes the birth of a new child into a family during the course of an open dependency case when the parent or caregiver has been determined to lack the protective capacity to safely care for the children in the home and has not substantially complied with the case plan toward successful reunification or met the conditions for return of the children into the home. Abuse of a child includes acts or omissions. Harm to a Child's Health or Welfare can occur when a person inflicts or allows to be inflicted upon the child physical, mental, or emotional injury. Such injury includes, but is not limited to, any of the following:

Continued

Table A.4 *Continued*

1. Willful acts that produce specific serious injuries
2. Purposely gives a child poison, alcohol, drugs, or other substances that substantially affect the child's behavior, motor coordination, or judgment or that result in sickness or internal injury
3. Leaves a child without adult supervision or arrangement appropriate for the child's age or mental or physical condition
4. Uses inappropriate or excessively harsh discipline that is likely to result in physical injury, mental injury as defined in this section, or emotional injury
5. Commits or allows to be committed sexual battery against the child
6. Allows, encourages, or forces the sexual exploitation of a child
7. Abandons the child
8. Exploits a child or allows a child to be exploited
9. Neglects the child
10. Exposes a child to a controlled substance or alcohol
11. Uses mechanical devices, unreasonable restraints, or extended periods of isolation to control a child
12. Engages in violent behavior that demonstrates a wanton disregard for the presence of a child and could reasonably result in serious injury to the child
13. Negligently fails to protect a child in his or her care from inflicted physical, mental, or sexual injury caused by the acts of another
14. Has allowed a child's sibling to die as a result of abuse, abandonment, or neglect
15. Makes the child unavailable for the purpose of impeding or avoiding a protective investigation unless the court determines that the parent, legal custodian, or caregiver was fleeing from a situation involving domestic violence

Exceptions: Corporal Discipline of a child by a parent or legal custodian for disciplinary purposes does not in itself constitute abuse when it does not result in harm to the child.

Georgia Child Abuse means physical injury or death inflicted upon a child by a parent or caregiver by other than accidental means.

Exceptions: Physical forms of discipline may be used as long as there is no physical injury to the child.

Kentucky Abused or Neglected Child means a child whose health or welfare is harmed or threatened with harm when his or her parent, guardian, or other person exercising custodial control or supervision does either of the following:
1. Inflicts or allows to be inflicted upon the child physical or emotional injury by other than accidental means
2. Creates or allows to be created a risk of physical or emotional injury to the child by other than accidental means

Physical Injury means substantial physical pain or any impairment of physical condition.

Serious Physical Injury means physical injury that creates a substantial risk of death or causes serious and prolonged disfigurement, prolonged impairment of health, or prolonged loss or impairment of the function of any bodily member or organ.

Table A.4 *Continued*

Louisiana	Abuse means any one of the following acts that seriously endanger the physical, mental, or emotional health and safety of the child:

Louisiana

Abuse means any one of the following acts that seriously endanger the physical, mental, or emotional health and safety of the child:

1. The infliction; attempted infliction; or, as a result of inadequate supervision, the allowance of the infliction or attempted infliction of physical or mental injury upon the child by a parent or any other person
2. Exploitation or overwork of a child by a parent or any other person, including, but not limited to, commercial sexual exploitation of the child
3. A coerced abortion conducted upon a child

The term Crime Against the Child shall include the commission of or the attempted commission of any of the following crimes against the child as provided by Federal or State statutes:

1. Homicide
2. Assault or battery
3. Kidnapping
4. Criminal neglect
5. Cruelty to juveniles
6. Contributing to the delinquency or dependency of children
7. Sale of minor children
8. Human trafficking

Maryland

Abuse means either of the following:

1. The physical or mental injury of a child under circumstances that indicate that the child's health or welfare is harmed or at substantial risk of being harmed by any of the following:
   a. A parent
   b. A household member or family member
   c. A person who has permanent or temporary care or custody of the child
   d. A person who has responsibility for supervision of the child
   e. A person who, because of the person's position or occupation, exercises authority over the child
2. Sexual abuse of a child, whether physical injuries are sustained or not

Abuse does not include the physical injury of a child by accidental means.

Mississippi

Abused Child means a child whose parent, guardian, custodian, or any person responsible for his or her care or support, whether or not legally obligated to do so, has caused or allowed to be caused upon the child nonaccidental physical injury or other maltreatment. The term abused child also means a child who is or has been trafficked within the meaning of the Mississippi Human Trafficking Act by any person, without regard to the relationship of the person to the child.

Exceptions: Physical discipline, including spanking, performed on a child by a parent, guardian, or custodian in a reasonable manner shall not be deemed abuse under this section.

North Carolina

Abused Juvenile means any child younger than age 18 who is found to be a minor victim of human trafficking under §14-43.15 or whose parent, guardian, custodian, or caregiver does any of the following:

1. Inflicts or allows to be inflicted upon the child a serious physical injury by other than accidental means
2. Creates or allows to be created a substantial risk of serious physical injury to the child by other than accidental means
3. Uses or allows to be used upon the child cruel or grossly inappropriate procedures or cruel or grossly inappropriate devices to modify behavior
4. Encourages, directs, or approves of delinquent acts involving moral turpitude committed by the juvenile

Continued

Table A.4 *Continued*

	5. Commits or allows to be committed the offense of human trafficking, involuntary servitude, or sexual servitude against the child
	This term includes any juvenile younger than age 18 who is a victim or is alleged to be a victim of human trafficking, involuntary servitude, or sexual servitude, regardless of the relationship between the victim and the perpetrator.
Oklahoma	Abuse means harm or threatened harm to the health, safety, or welfare of a child by a person responsible for the child's health, safety, or welfare, including, but not limited to, nonaccidental physical or mental injury, sexual abuse, or sexual exploitation.
	Harm or Threatened Harm to the Health or Safety of a Child means any real or threatened physical, mental, or emotional injury or damage to the body or mind that is not accidental, including, but not limited to, sexual abuse, sexual exploitation, neglect, or dependency.
	Heinous and Shocking Abuse includes, but is not limited to, aggravated physical abuse that results in serious bodily, mental, or emotional injury.
	Serious Bodily Injury means injury that involves any of the following: 1. A substantial risk of death 2. Extreme physical pain 3. Protracted disfigurement 4. A loss or impairment of the function of a body member, organ, or mental faculty 5. An injury to an internal or external organ or the body 6. A bone fracture 7. Sexual abuse or sexual exploitation 8. Chronic abuse, including, but not limited to, physical, emotional, or sexual abuse, or sexual exploitation that is repeated or continuing 9. Torture, including, but not limited to, inflicting, participating in, or assisting in inflicting intense physical or emotional pain upon a child repeatedly over a period of time for the purpose of coercing or terrorizing a child for the purpose of satisfying the craven, cruel, or prurient desires of the perpetrator or another person 10. Any other similar aggravated circumstance
	Exceptions: Nothing contained in this act shall prohibit any parent, teacher, or other person from using ordinary force as a means of discipline, including, but not limited to, spanking, switching, or paddling.

South Carolina	Child Abuse or Neglect or Harm occurs under the following circumstances:
	1. The parent, guardian, or other person responsible for the child's welfare does any of the following:
	  a. Inflicts or allows to be inflicted upon the child physical or mental injury or engages in acts or omissions that present a substantial risk of physical or mental injury to the child, including injuries sustained as a result of excessive corporal punishment
	  b. Abandons the child
	  c. Encourages, condones, or approves the commission of delinquent acts by the child, and the commission of the acts are shown to be the result of the encouragement or approval
	  d. Has committed abuse or neglect, as described above, such that a child who subsequently becomes part of the person's household is at substantial risk of one of those forms of abuse or neglect
	2. A child is a victim of trafficking in persons, as defined in §16-3-2010, including sex trafficking, regardless of whether the perpetrator is a parent, guardian, or other person responsible for the child's welfare. Identifying a child as a victim of trafficking in persons does not create a presumption that the parent, guardian, or other individual responsible for the child's welfare abused, neglected, or harmed the child.

Table A.4 *Continued*

Physical Injury means death or permanent or temporary disfigurement or impairment of any bodily organ or function.

Exceptions: The term Child Abuse or Neglect excludes corporal punishment or physical discipline that consists of the following:
1. Is administered by a parent or person in loco parentis
2. Is perpetrated for the sole purpose of restraining or correcting the child
3. Is reasonable in manner and moderate in degree
4. Has not brought about permanent or lasting damage to the child
5. Is not reckless or grossly negligent behavior by the parents

Tennessee	Abuse exists when a person under age 18 is suffering from, has sustained, or may be in immediate danger of suffering from or sustaining a wound, injury, disability, or physical or mental condition caused by brutality, neglect, or other actions or inactions of a parent, relative, guardian, or caregiver.

Severe Child Abuse means any of the following:
1. The knowing exposure of a child to, or the knowing failure to protect a child from, abuse or neglect that is likely to cause serious bodily injury or death and the knowing use of force on a child that is likely to cause serious bodily injury
2. Specific brutality, abuse, or neglect toward a child that, in the opinion of qualified experts, has caused or will reasonably be expected to produce severe psychosis, severe neurotic disorder, severe depression, severe developmental delay or retardation, or severe impairment of the child's ability to function adequately in the child's environment and the knowing failure to protect a child from such conduct
3. The commission of any act toward the child prohibited by §§39-13-309 (trafficking for a commercial sex act), 39-13-502 (aggravated rape), 39-13-503 (rape), 39-13-504 (aggravated sexual battery), 39-13-515 (promoting prostitution), 39-13-522 (rape of a child), 39-15-302 (incest), 39-15-402 (aggravated child abuse, neglect, or endangerment), and 39-17-1005 (aggravated sexual exploitation of a minor) or the knowing failure to protect the child from the commission of any such act towards the child
4. Knowingly allowing a child to be present within a structure where the act of creating methamphetamine is occurring

Significant Injury means bodily injury, including a cut, abrasion, bruise, burn, or disfigurement, and physical pain or temporary illness or impairment of the function of a bodily member, organ, or mental faculty, involving any of the following:
1. A substantial risk of death
2. Protracted unconsciousness
3. Extreme physical pain
4. Protracted or obvious disfigurement
5. Protracted loss or substantial impairment of a function of a bodily member, organ, or mental faculty

Abuse means the following acts or omissions by a person:
1. Physical injury that results in substantial harm to the child or the genuine threat of substantial harm from physical injury to the child, including an injury that is inconsistent with the history or explanation given and excluding an accident or reasonable discipline by a parent, guardian, or conservator that does not expose the child to a substantial risk of harm
2. Failure to make a reasonable effort to prevent an action by another person that results in physical injury or substantial harm to the child
3. The current use by a person of a controlled substance in a manner or to the extent that the use results in physical, mental, or emotional injury to a child

Continued

Table A.4 *Continued*

Texas	4. Causing, expressly permitting, or encouraging a child to use a controlled substance
	5. Forcing or coercing a child to enter into a marriage

Exploitation means the illegal or improper use of a child or of the resources of a child for monetary or personal benefit, profit, or gain by an employee, volunteer, or other individual working under the auspices of a facility or program.

Exceptions: Abuse does not include reasonable discipline by a parent that does not expose the child to substantial risk of harm.

Virginia	Abused or Neglected Child means any child younger than age 18 whose parents or other person responsible for his or her care creates or inflicts, threatens to create or inflict, or allows to be created or inflicted upon the child a physical or mental injury by other than accidental means or creates a substantial risk of death, disfigurement, or impairment of bodily or mental functions, including, but not limited to, a child who is with his or her parent or other person responsible for his or her care either (i) during the manufacture or attempted manufacture of a Schedule I or II controlled substance or (ii) during the unlawful sale of such substance by that child's parents or other person responsible for his or her care, when such manufacture, or attempted manufacture, or unlawful sale would constitute a felony violation.
West Virginia	Abused Child means a child whose health or welfare is being harmed or threatened by any of the following:

1. A parent, guardian, or custodian who knowingly or intentionally inflicts, attempts to inflict, or knowingly allows another person to inflict, physical injury or mental or emotional injury upon the child or another child in the home, including an injury to the child as a result of excessive corporal punishment
2. Sexual abuse or sexual exploitation
3. The sale or attempted sale of a child by a parent, guardian, or custodian in violation of §61-2-14h
4. Domestic violence, as defined in §48-27-202
5. Human trafficking or attempted human trafficking in violation of §61-14-2

Imminent Danger to the Physical Well-being of the Child means an emergency situation in which the welfare or the life of the child is threatened. These conditions may include a situation when there is reasonable cause to believe that any child in the home is or has been sexually abused or sexually exploited or there is reasonable cause to believe that the following conditions threaten the health, life, or safety of any child in the home:

1. Nonaccidental trauma inflicted by a parent, guardian, custodian, sibling, babysitter, or other caregiver
2. A combination of physical and other signs indicating a pattern of abuse that may be medically diagnosed as battered child syndrome
3. Sale or attempted sale of the child by the parent, guardian, or custodian
4. Any other condition that threatens the health, life, or safety of any child in the home. Serious physical abuse means bodily injury that creates a substantial risk of death, or causes serious or prolonged disfigurement, prolonged impairment of health, or prolonged loss or impairment of the function of any bodily organ.

*Excludes independent sections on emotional, verbal, and sexual child abuse.

Source: Children's Bureau, Child Welfare Information Gateway, Definitions of Child Abuse and Neglect, State Statues Current through March 2019. https://www.childwelfare.gov/topics/systemwide/laws-policies/statutes/define/

Definition of School Corporal Punishment and Legal Language

State and Source	Definition of Corporal Punishment	Legal Language
Alabama http://alisondb.legislat ure.state.al.us/alison/ codeofalabama/1975/ coatoc.htm **Section 16-28A-1**	None	"The teacher in each classroom is expected to maintain order and discipline. Teachers are hereby given the authority and responsibility to use appropriate means of discipline up to and including corporal punishment as may be prescribed by the local board of education. So long as teachers follow approved policy in the exercise of their responsibility to maintain discipline in their classroom, such teacher shall be immune from civil or criminal liability."
Arizona https://www.azleg. gov/FormatDocum ent.asp?inDoc=/ars/ 15/00843.htm&Title= 15&DocType=ARS iabi15-843. Pupil disci-plinary proceedings	None	"The governing board of any school district, in consultation with the teachers and parents of the school district, shall prescribe rules for the discipline, suspension and expulsion of pupils. The rules shall be consistent with the constitutional rights of pupils and shall include at least the following: Procedures for the use of corporal punishment if allowed by the governing board."
Arkansas www.arkleg.state.ar.us/ acts/1993S2/Public/ 51.pdf	None	"A school district that authorizes use of corporal punishment in its discipline policy shall include provisions for administration of the punishment, including that it be administered only for cause, be reasonable, follow warnings that the misbehavior will not be tolerated, and be administered by a teacher or an administrator employed by the school district."
Colorado http://coddc.org/ Documents/CO%20 Statutes%20-- %20Care%20and%20 Treatment%20 of%20the%20 Developmentally%20 Disabled.pdf	None	"Corporal punishment of persons with a developmental disability shall not be permitted."

Continued

State and Source	Definition of Corporal Punishment	Legal Language
Florida www.leg.state. fl.us/Statutes/ index.cfm?App_ mode=Display_ Statute&Search_String= &URL=1000-1099/ 1003/Sections/1003.32. html	None	"The use of corporal punishment shall be approved in principle by the principal before it is used, but approval is not necessary for each specific instance in which it is used. The principal shall prepare guidelines for administering such punishment which identify the types of punishable offenses, the conditions under which the punishment shall be administered, and the specific personnel on the school staff authorized to administer the punishment."
Georgia http://ga.elaws.us/law/ section20-2-731	None	"An area, county, or independent board of education may, upon the adoption of written policies, authorize any principal or teacher employed by the board to administer, in the exercise of his sound discretion, corporal punishment on any pupil or pupils placed under his supervision in order to maintain proper control and discipline. Any such authorization shall be subject to the following requirements: 1) The corporal punishment shall not be excessive or unduly severe; (2) Corporal punishment shall never be used as a first line of punishment for misbehavior unless the pupil was informed beforehand that specific misbehavior could occasion its use."
Idaho https://legislature.idaho. gov/statutesrules/idstat/ Title33/T33CH12/ SECT33-1224/	None	"It is the duty of a teacher to carry out the rules and regulations of the board of trustees in controlling and maintaining discipline, and a teacher shall have the power to adopt any reasonable rule or regulation to control and maintain discipline in, and otherwise govern, the classroom, not inconsistent with any statute or rule or regulation of the board of trustees."
Indiana https://statelaws.findlaw. com/indiana-law/ indiana-corporal- punishment-in-public- schools-laws.ht	None	
Kansas http://www.kansas. com/news/politics- government/ar- ticle1134733.html	None	

State and Source	Definition of Corporal Punishment	Legal Language
Kentucky http://www.lrc.ky.gov/ statutes/statute.aspx?id= 19677	None	"The use of physical force by a defendant upon another person is justifiable when the defendant is a parent, guardian, or other person entrusted with the care and supervision of a minor or an incompetent person or when the defendant is a teacher or other person entrusted with the care and supervision of a minor, or mentally disabled person is for a special purpose, to further that special purpose or maintain reasonable discipline in a school, class, or other group; and (b) The force that is used is not designed to cause or known to create a substantial risk of causing death, serious physical injury, disfigurement, extreme pain, or extreme mental distress. "
Louisiana http://www.legis.la.gov/ legis/law.aspx?d=81025	"Corporal punishment means using physical force to discipline a student, with or without an object. Corporal punishment includes hitting, paddling, striking, spanking, slapping, or any other physical force that causes pain or physical discomfort. (i) The use of reasonable and necessary physical restraint of a student to protect the student, or others, from bodily harm or to obtain possession of a weapon or other dangerous object from a student."	"The governing authority of a public elementary or secondary school shall have discretion with respect to the use of corporal punishment; however, no form of corporal punishment shall be administered to a student with an exceptionality, excluding gifted and talented, as defined in R.S. 17:1942 or to a student who has been determined to be eligible for services under Section 504 of the Rehabilitation Act of 1973 and has an Individual Accommodation Plan."
Mississippi https://statepolicies. nasbe.org/health/ categories/physical- environment/corporal- punishment/mississippi	"For the purposes of this subsection, 'corporal punishment' means the reasonable use of physical force or physical contact by a teacher, assistant teacher, principal or assistant principal, as may be necessary to maintain discipline, to enforce a school rule, for self-protection or for the protection of other students from disruptive students."	"Corporal punishment administered in a reasonable manner, or any reasonable action to maintain control and discipline of students taken by a public school teacher, assistant teacher, principal or assistant principal acting within the scope of his employment or function and in accordance with any state or federal laws or rules or regulations of the State Board of Education or the local school board or governing board of a charter school does not constitute negligence or child abuse."

Continued

State and Source	Definition of Corporal Punishment	Legal Language
Missouri http://revisor.mo.gov/ main/OneSection. aspx?section= 160.261&bid=7750&hl=	None	"Spanking, when administered by certificated personnel and in the presence of a witness who is an employee of the school district, or the use of reasonable force to protect persons or property, when administered by personnel of a school district in a reasonable manner in accordance with the local board of education's written policy of discipline, is not abuse within the meaning of chapter 210."
North Carolina https://www.ncleg.net/ enactedlegislation/ statutes/pdf/bysection/ chapter_115c/gs_ 115c-390.4.pdf	"[S]chool personnel may use physical restraint in accordance with federal law and G.S. 115C-391.1 and reasonable force pursuant to G.S. 115C-390.3."	"Each local board of education shall determine whether corporal punishment will be permitted in its school administrative unit. Notwithstanding a local board of education's prohibition on the use of corporal punishment, school personnel may use physical restraint in accordance with federal law and G.S. 115C-391.1 and reasonable force pursuant to G.S. 115C-390.3."
Oklahoma https://law.justia. com/codes/okla- homa/2014/title-70/ section-70-24-100.4/	None	"The teacher of a child attending a public school shall have the same right as a parent or guardian to control and discipline such child according to district policies during the time the child is in attendance or in transit to or from the school or any other school function authorized by the school district or classroom presided over by the teacher."
South Carolina http://www. scstatehouse.gov/code/ t59c063.php	None	"The governing body of each school district may provide corporal punishment for any pupil that it deems just and proper."
Tennessee https:// safesupportivelearning. ed.gov/sites/default/ files/discipline- compendium/ Tennessee%20 School%20 Discipline%20Laws%20 and%20Regulations.pdf	None	"Any teacher or school principal may use corporal punishment in a reasonable manner against any pupil for good cause in order to maintain discipline and order within the public schools."

State and Source	Definition of Corporal Punishment	Legal Language
Texas https://statutes.capitol. texas.gov/Docs/ED/ htm/ED.37.htm#37.0011	"[T]he deliberate infliction of physical pain by hitting, paddling, spanking, slapping, or any other physical force used as a means of discipline. The term does not include: 1) physical pain caused by reasonable physical activities associated with athletic training, competition, or physical education; or the use of restraint as authorized under Section 37.0021."	"If the board of trustees of an independent school district adopts a policy under Section 37.001(a)(8) under which corporal punishment is permitted as a method of student discipline, a district educator may use corporal punishment to discipline a student unless the student's parent or guardian or other person having lawful control over the student has previously provided a written, signed statement prohibiting the use of corporal punishment as a method of student discipline."
Wyoming http://legisweb.state. wy.us/NXT/gateway. dll?f=templates&fn= default.htm	None	"Each board of trustees in each school district within the state may adopt rules for reasonable forms of punishment and disciplinary measures. Subject to such rules, teachers, principals, and superintendents in such district may impose reasonable forms of punishment and disciplinary measures for insubordination, disobedience, and other misconduct. Teachers, principals and superintendents in each district shall be immune from civil and criminal liability in the exercise of reasonable corporal discipline of a student as authorized by board policy."

School Corporal Punishment Administration and Required Parental Communication

State	Who Monitors	Who Can Administer	Parental Communication
Alabama	Local board of education	Public school teachers or other employees in the classroom and on public school property, including school buses	Each local board of education must distribute their policy on student discipline and behavior to all teachers, staff, parents, and students.
Arizona	Governing board of the school district	Not specified	None required
Arkansas	School district board	Persons employed by a school district and required to have a state-issued license	None required
Colorado	Not specified	Not specified	None required
Florida	School district board, and then school principal (except in certain circumstances)	Teacher or principals and only in the presence of another adult who is informed beforehand	Parents may request a written explanation of the reason for the corporal punishment from the teacher or principal who administered it and the name of the other adult who was present.
Georgia	Area, county, and independent boards of education	Any principal or teacher employed by the board	A student may not be corporally punished if parent or guardian can provide a statement from a medical doctor licensed in Georgia that states that corporal punishment may be damaging to the student's mental or emotional well-being. Parents may also request information regarding incidents of corporal punishment after the student has received it.
Idaho	District board of trustees	Teacher employed by a school district	None required
Indiana	Not specified	Not specified	None required
Kansas	Not specified	Not specified	None required
Kentucky	Local school districts	Teachers	None required

State	Who Monitors	Who Can Administer	Parental Communication
Louisiana	The governing authority of a public elementary or secondary school	Teachers, principals, and administrators of the public schools	None required
Mississippi	State board of education or the local school board or governing board of a charter school	Public school teacher, assistant teacher, principal, or assistant principal	None required
Missouri	Local board of education in each school district	"Certificated personnel"	A copy of the school district's disciple and corporal punishment policy and procedures is provided to parent or legal guardian at the beginning of the school year.
North Carolina	Local board of education	Teacher, principal, or assistant principal in the presence of a principal, assistant principal, or teacher	Corporal punishment is not administered to students whose parent or guardian has provided a written statement that corporal punishment shall not be administered to their child. Parents and guardians receive a notification when corporal punishment is administered, and the person who administered the punishment will provide a written explanation of reasoning and the name of the other adult present.
Oklahoma	District board of education	Teachers	Parents and guardians will be notified upon the adoption of the district's policy and can request a copy.
South Carolina	Governing body of school district	Not specified	None required
Tennessee	Local board of education	The chief administrative officer, or the chief administrative officer's designee, only in a classroom situation and in the presence of one other faculty	None required
Texas	Board of trustees in an independent school district	District educator	A student will not receive corporal punishment if their parent or guardian provides a written and signed statement. A new statement must be provided every school year.
Wyoming	Board of trustees in a school district	Teachers, principals, and superintendents	None required

Bans on Physical Punishment of Children: Year and Country

Year Banned	Country
2021	Republic of Korea, Colombia
2020	Japan, Seychelles, Guinea
2019	Georgia, South Africa, France, Republic of Kosovo
2018	Nepal
2017	Lithuania
2016	Mongolia, Montenegro, Paraguay, Slovenia
2015	Benin, Ireland, Peru
2014	Andorra, Estonia, Nicaragua, San Marino, Argentina, Bolivia, Brazil, Malta
2013	Cabo Verde, Honduras, North Macedonia
2012	South Sudan
2010	Albania, Congo (Republic of), Kenya, Tunisia, Poland
2008	Liechtenstein, Luxembourg, Republic of Moldova, Costa Rica
2007	Togo, Spain, Venezuela, Uruguay, Portugal, New Zealand, Netherlands
2006	Greece
2005	Hungary
2004	Romania, Ukraine
2003	Iceland
2002	Turkmenistan
2000	Germany, Israel, Bulgaria
1999	Croatia
1998	Latvia
1997	Denmark
1994	Cyprus
1989	Austria
1987	Norway
1983	Finland
1979	Sweden

Source: Global Initiative to End All Corporal Punishment of Children. https://endcorporalpunishment.org/countdown/

Policy Language of National Bans on Physical Punishment

Year Banned	Country	Legal Language
2021	Republic of Korea	The protector of children (i.e., parents and other adults with parental authority) "shall rear the children healthy and safely within the family, according to the stage of their growth" and all citizens "shall respect the rights, interests and safety of children and rear them healthy." A protector shall not "inflict physical pain or psychological pain, including violent language, on the children."
2021	Colombia	"Parents or individuals who exercise parental authority over children and adolescents have the right to educate, raise and correct their children according to their beliefs and values. The only limit is the prohibition to use physical punishment, cruel, humiliating, or degrading treatment and any type of violence against children and adolescents. The prohibition extends to any other person responsible for their care, in each of the different environments where childhood and adolescence unfold."
2020	Japan	"A person who exercises parental authority over a child shall not discipline the child by inflicting corporal punishment upon him/her or by taking other forms of action that go beyond the scope necessary for the care and education of the child . . . and shall give due consideration to appropriate exercise of parental authority over the child."
2020	Seychelles	"Notwithstanding any other law, no child shall be subjected to corporal punishment."
2019	Georgia	"Corporal punishment, torture or any other cruel, degrading or inhuman treatment or punishment of children shall be prohibited in the family, preschool or general education institutions, alternative care services, medical and/or psychiatric institutions, penitentiary facilities and any other places. The commission of such acts shall be punishable under the effective legislation of Georgia."
	South Africa	"[T]o inflict moderate and reasonable chastisement on a child for misconduct provided that this was not done in a manner offensive to good morals or for objects other than correction and admonition under South Africa's common law system, this decision from the Constitutional Court is equivalent to repealing the defence in legislation. With this decision, the Court effectively banned the use of all corporal punishment in the home, as criminal provisions against assault now apply equally to children."

Continued

Year Banned	Country	Legal Language
	France	"Parental authority is exercised without any physical or psychological violence."
	Republic of Kosovo	"Child attending all forms of pre-university education is protected from all types of violence, abuse, exploitation, corporal punishment, neglecting or any other form that puts at risk his/her life, safety, health, education and development of the child by the educational personnel, by their peers and any other person within the educational system while conducting the activities."
2018	Nepal	"Each child has a right to be protected against all types of physical or mental violence and punishment, neglect, inhumane behaviour, gender based or discriminatory abuse, sexual abuse and exploitation committed by his/her father, mother, other family members or guardian, teacher or any other person."
2017	Lithuania	"Parents and other legal representatives of the child may appropriately, according to their judgment, discipline the child, for avoiding to carry out his duties and for disciplinary infractions, with the exception of corporal punishment and any other form of violence."
2016	Mongolia	"All types of physical and humiliating punishment against children by parents, guardians and third parties who are responsible for care, treatment, guidance and education of children and adolescents, during the upbringing and disciplining faulty behaviours of children is prohibited."
	Montenegro	"Child shall not be subjected to corporal punishment or any other cruel, inhuman or degrading treatment. The prohibition referred to in para 1 above shall pertain to parents, guardians and all other persons taking care of or coming into contact with the child. The persons referred to in para 2 above are obliged to protect the child from any treatment referred to in para 1 above."
	Paraguay	"All children and adolescents have the right to good treatment and for their physical, psychological and emotional integrity to be respected. This right includes the protection of their image, their identity, their autonomy, their thoughts, their feelings, their dignity and their values. Corporal punishment and humiliating treatment of children and adolescents is prohibited as a form of correction or discipline, especially when it is imparted by parents, tutors, guardians or anyone responsible for their education, care, guidance, or treatment of any kind. Children and adolescents are especially entitled to receive guidance, education, care and discipline by implementing guidelines for positive parenting."
	Slovenia	"Corporal punishment of children is prohibited. Corporal punishment of children is any physical, cruel or degrading punishment of children or any other act with the intention to punish children, containing elements of physical, psychological or sexual violence or neglect as an educational method."

Year Banned	Country	Legal Language
2015	Benin	"Parents or other persons legally responsible for a child will ensure that discipline is enforced in such a way as to ensure that it is treated with humanity and with respect for its human dignity. If necessary, they may punish the child. In no case may the punishment constitute a violation of the child's physical integrity or torture or inhuman or degrading treatment. Any punishment must be educational in intent and accompanied by an explanation."
	Ireland	"The common law defence of reasonable chastisement is abolished. . . ."
	Peru	"Purpose of the Law. To prohibit the use of physical and humiliating punishment against children and adolescents. This prohibition applies in all areas where children and adolescents are, including the home, school, community, workplaces and other related places."
2014	Andorra	"Whoever corporally mistreats mildly or harms physically, a person, shall be punished by imprisonment or a fine up to 6.000 euros. If the mistreatment consists of a corporal punishment, a sentence of imprisonment shall be imposed."
	Estonia	"It is prohibited to neglect a child, to mentally, emotionally, physically or sexually abuse a child, including to humiliate, frighten or physically punish a child, and also to punish a child in any other way that endangers the mental, emotional or physical health of a child. . . ."
	Nicaragua	"The father, mother, or other family members, guardians or other persons legally responsible for the son or daughter have the responsibility, the right and duty to provide, consistent with the child's evolving capacities, appropriate direction and guidance to the child, without putting at risk his or her health, physical integrity, psychological and personal dignity and under no circumstances using physical punishment or any type of humiliating treatment as a form of correction or discipline."
	San Marino	"Children have the right to protection and security, and shall not be subjected to corporal punishment or other treatment harmful to their physical and psychological integrity."
	Argentina	"All forms of corporal punishment, ill-treatment and any act that physically or mentally injures or impairs children and adolescents are prohibited. . . ."
	Bolivia	"Right to good treatment. The child and adolescent has the right to good treatment, comprising a non-violent upbringing and education, based on mutual respect and solidarity. The exercise of the authority of the mother, father, guardian, family members and educators should use non-violent methods in parenting, education and correction. Any physical, violent and humiliating punishment is prohibited."
	Brazil	"Children and adolescents are entitled to be educated and cared for without the use of physical punishment or cruel or degrading treatment as forms of correction, discipline, education or any other pretext, by their parents, by the members of their extended family, by persons responsible for them, by public officials implementing social and educational measures or by any other person entrusted with taking care of them or treating, educating or protecting them. . . ."

Continued

Year Banned	Country	Legal Language
	Malta	"Provided that, for the avoidance of any doubt, corporal punishment of any kind shall always be deemed to exceed the bounds of moderation."
2013	Cabo Verde	"The family must provide a loving and safe environment that allows the full development of children and adolescents and protects them from any actions affecting their personal integrity. In exercising the right to correction parents must always keep in mind the rights of children and adolescents to an upbringing free from violence, corporal punishment, psychological harm and any other measures affecting their dignity, which are all inadmissible."
	Honduras	"Parents, in the exercise of parental authority, have the right to exercise orientation, care and correction of their children, and to import to them, in keeping with the evolution of their physical and mental faculties, the guidance and orientation which are appropriate for their comprehensive development. It is prohibited to parents and every person charged with the care, upbringing, education, treatment and monitoring [of children and adolescents], whether on a temporary or permanent basis, to use physical punishment or any type of humiliating, degrading, cruel or inhuman treatment as a form of correction or discipline of children or adolescents."
	North Macedonia	"All forms of sexual exploitation and sexual child abuse (harassment, child pornography, child prostitution), forced procuring, selling or trafficking children, psychological or physical violence and harassment, punishment or other inhuman treatment, all kinds of exploitation, commercial exploitation and abuse of children that violates basic human freedoms and rights and rights of the child, are prohibited."
2011	South Sudan	"Every child has the right . . . to be free from corporal punishment and cruel and inhuman treatment by any person including parents, school administrations and other institutions. . . ."
2010	Albania	"Corporal punishment or punishment of any other form entailing consequences on the physical and mental development of the child shall be prohibited." Corporal punishment is defined as: "any form of punishment in which physical force is used and intended to cause pain or discomfort to the child, by any person who is legally responsible for the child. Corporal punishment includes the following forms: smacking, torturing, shaking, pushing, burning, slapping, pinching, scratching, biting, scolding, pulling the hair, forcing an action, using substances that cause pain or discomfort as well as any other similar act."
	Republic of Congo	"It is forbidden to use corporal punishment to discipline or correct the child."
	Kenya	"[T]he right to freedom and security of the person, which includes the right not to be . . . (c) subjected to any form of violence from either public or private sources; (d) subjected to torture in any manner, whether physical or psychological; (e) subjected to corporal punishment; or (f) treated or punished in a cruel, inhuman or degrading manner."

Year Banned	Country	Legal Language
	Tunisia	"Children are guaranteed the rights to dignity, health, care and education from their parents and the state. The state must provide all types of protection to all children without discrimination and in accordance with their best interest."
	Poland	"Persons who exercise parental authority and who provide care of or custody over a minor may not apply corporal punishment."
2008	Liechtenstein	"(1) Children and young people have the rights outlined in the Convention on the Rights of the Child and to the following measures: (a) protection notably against discrimination, neglect, violence, abuse and sexual abuse; (b) education/upbringing without violence: corporal punishment, psychological harm and other degrading treatment are not accepted. . . . (2) Children can address the Ombudsperson when they believe their rights have been violated."
	Luxembourg	Prohibits physical violence and inhuman and degrading treatment within families and educative communities, and this is interpreted as prohibiting all corporal punishment, however light, in the home
	Republic of Moldova	Confirm the right of the child "to be protected against abuse, including corporal punishment by his parents or persons who replace them"
	Costa Rica	"Parental authority confers the rights and imposes the duties to orient, educate, care, supervise and discipline the children, which in no case authorises the use of corporal punishment or any other form of degrading treatment against the minors. . . ."
2007	Togo	"The state protects the child from all forms of violence including sexual abuse, physical or mental injury or abuse, abandonment or neglect, and ill treatment by parents or by any other person having control or custody over him." "Physical and psychological abuse, corporal punishment, deprivation of care or withholding of food are punished by the penalties provided [above]."
	Spain	Parents/guardians must exercise their authority with respect for the child's physical and psychological integrity.
	Venezuela	"The responsibility for raising children includes the shared duty and right, which is equal and non-derogable, of the father and mother to love, raise, train, educate, and look after their children, sustain and assist them financially, morally and emotionally, using appropriate corrective measures that do not violate their dignity, rights, guarantees or overall development. Consequently, all forms of physical punishment, psychological violence and humiliating treatment, which harm children and young people, are prohibited."
	Uruguay	"Prohibition of corporal punishment. Parents and guardians, as well as all persons responsible for the care, treatment, education or supervision of children and adolescents, are prohibited from using corporal punishment or any type of humiliating treatment as a means of reprimanding or disciplining them."
	Portugal	"Whoever repeatedly, or not, inflicts physical or psychological ill-treatment, including corporal punishment, deprivation of liberty and sexual offences, is punished with 1 to 5 years of imprisonment."

Continued

Year Banned	Country	Legal Language
	New Zealand	"[N]othing in subsection (1) or in any rule of common law justifies the use of force for the purpose of correction."
	Netherlands	"(1) Parental authority includes the duty and the right of the parent to care for and raise his or her minor child. (2) Caring for and raising one's child includes the care and the responsibility for the emotional and physical wellbeing of the child and for his or her safety as well as for the promotion of the development of his or her personality. In the care and upbringing of the child the parents will not use emotional or physical violence or any other humiliating treatment."
2006	Greece	"Physical violence against children as a disciplinary measure in the context of their upbringing brings the consequences of Article 1532 of the Civil Code."
2005	Hungary	"The child has the right to respect of his/her human dignity, to be protected against abuse—physical, sexual and mental violence—failure to provide care and injury caused by any information. The child shall not be subjected to torture, corporal punishment and any cruel, inhuman or degrading punishment or treatment."
2004	Romania	"It is forbidden to enforce physical punishment of any kind or to deprive the child of his or her rights, which may result in endangerment of the life, the physical, mental, spiritual, moral and social development, the bodily integrity, and the physical and mental health of the child, both within the family as well as in any institutions which ensures the protection, care and education of children."
	Ukraine	"Every child is guaranteed the right to liberty, personal security and dignity. Discipline and order in the family, education and other children's facilities should be provided on the principles based on mutual respect, justice and without humiliation of the honour and dignity of the child. . . ."
2003	Iceland	"Any person who inflicts punishments, threats or menaces upon a child, that may be expected to harm the child physically or mentally, is subject to fines or imprisonment for up to three years."
2002	Turkmenistan	"When implementing parental rights, parents shall not do injury (harm) to the physical and mental health of the child, its moral development. Methods of education shall exclude neglectful, cruel . . . degrading treatment. . . ."
2000	Germany	"[Family support measures] should help to ensure that mothers, fathers and other guardians carry out their parental responsibilities better. They should also identify ways in which conflict situations in the family can be resolved without violence."

Year Banned	Country	Legal Language
	Israel	"Accordingly, we decide that corporal punishment of children, or humiliation and derogation from their dignity as a method of education by their parents, is entirely impermissible, and is a remnant of a societal-educational outlook that has lost its validity. The child is not the parent's property and cannot be used as a punching bag the parents can beat at their leisure, even when the parents honestly believe that they are fulfilling their duty and right to educate their child. The child depends upon the parents, is entitled to parental love, protection and the parents' gentle touch. The use of punishment which causes hurt and humiliation does not contribute to the child's personality or education, but instead damages his or her human rights. Such punishment injures his or her body, feelings, dignity and proper development. Such punishment distances us from our goal of a society free of violence. Accordingly, let it be known that in our society, parents are now forbidden to make use of corporal punishments or methods that demean and humiliate the child as an educational system."
	Bulgaria	"Every child has a right to protection against all methods of upbringing that undermine his or her dignity; against physical, psychical or other types of violence; against all forms of influence, which go against his or her interests."
1999	Croatia	"Parents and other family members must not subject the child to degrading treatment, mental or physical punishment and abuse."
1998	Latvia	"A child cannot be treated cruelly, cannot be tormented and physically punished, and his/her dignity and honour cannot be offended."
1997	Denmark	The child "may not be subjected to corporal punishment or any other degrading treatment."
1994	Cyprus	"Any unlawful act or controlling behaviour which results in direct actual physical, sexual or psychological injury to any member of the family."
1989	Austria	"The minor child must follow the parents' orders. In their orders and in the implementation thereof, parents must consider the age, development and personality of the child; the use of force and infliction of physical or psychological suffering are not permitted."
1987	Norway	"The child must not be subjected to violence or in any other way be treated so as to harm or endanger his or her mental or physical health. This shall also apply when violence is carried out in connection with upbringing of the child. Use of violence and frightening or annoying behaviour or other inconsiderate conduct towards the child is prohibited."

Continued

Year Banned	Country	Legal Language
1983	Finland	"A child shall be brought up in the spirit of understanding, security and love. He shall not be subdued, corporally punished or otherwise humiliated. His growth towards independence, responsibility and adulthood shall be encouraged, supported and assisted."
1979	Sweden	"Children are entitled to care, security and a good upbringing. Children shall be treated with respect for their person and individuality and may not be subjected to corporal punishment or any other humiliating treatment."

Source: Global Initiative to End All Corporal Punishment of Children. https://endcorporalpunishment.org/reports-on-every-state-and-territory/
Some are unofficial translations to English.

Notes

Dedication

1. Kennedy, E. (1974). *Living with Everyday Problems*. Chicago, IL: Thomas More Press.

Preface

1. The General Social Survey (GSS) is a project of the independent research organization, NORC, at the University of Chicago, with principal funding from the National Science Foundation. https://gssdataexplorer.norc.org
2. Loseke, D. R., & Best, J. (2003). *Social Problems: Constructionist Readings*. Hawthorne, NY: Aldine DeGruyter.
3. Davis, P. W. (2003). The changing meanings of spanking. In Loseke, D. R. Loseke & J. Best. (Eds.), *Social Problems: Constructionist Readings* (pp. 3–12). Hawthorne, NY: Aldine DeGruyter.
4. Brown, B. (2012). *Daring Greatly: How the Courage to be Vulnerable Transforms the Way We Live, Love, Parent, and Lead* (p. 214). New York: Gotham.

Chapter 1

1. Cable, M. (1975). *The Little Darlings: A History of Child Rearing in America*. New York: Charles Scribner's Sons.
2. Robbins, M. (2014, September 15). Spanking isn't parenting: It's child abuse. *CNN Opinion*. http://www.cnn.com/2014/09/15/opinion/robbins-spanking-adrian-peterson-case/index.html
3. Pingleton, J. (2014, September 16). Spanking can be an appropriate form of discipline. *Time*. http://time.com/3387226/spanking-can-be-an-appropriate-form-of-child-discipline/
4. Sorkin, A. D. (2014, September 15). Adrian Peterson's intent. *The New Yorker*. https://www.newyorker.com/news/amy-davidson/adrian-petersons-intent
5. Gardner, S. (2018, November 21). Redskins' Adrian Peterson admits he still spanks his kids, even after 2014 NFL suspension. *USA Today*. https://www.usatoday.com/story/sports/nfl/redskins/2018/11/21/redskins-adrian-peterson-interview-still-spanks-children-nfl/2082957002/
6. *The Oprah Winfrey Show*. (1994, May). Hitting, spanking, slapping. https://www.youtube.com/watch?v=9T_4DgQ3fQM
7. Simons, D. A., & Wurtele, S. K. (2010). Relationships between parents' use of corporal punishment and their children's endorsement of spanking and hitting other children. *Child Abuse & Neglect, 34*(9), 639–646.

8. Nehandra Radio. (2014, September 21). Adrian Peterson controversy: To spank or not to spank? http://nehandaradio.com/2014/09/21/adrian-peterson-controversy-to-spank-or-not-to-spank/

9. English Language & Usage, Stack Exchange. https://english.stackexchange.com/questions/411065/why-isnt-it-corporeal-punishment-instead-of-corporal-punishment/411073#411073

10. Online Etymology Dictionary. https://www.etymonline.com/word/spank

11. English, Oxford Living Dictionaries. https://en.oxforddictionaries.com/definition/us/whup

12. Brown, A. S., Holden, G. W., & Ashraf, R. (2018). Spank, slap, or hit? How labels alter perceptions of child discipline. *Psychology of Violence, 8*(1), 1–9.

13. Straus, M. A., Gelles, R. J., & Steinmetz, S. K. (1980). *Behind Closed Doors: Violence in the American Family*. New York: Anchor Books.

14. General Social Survey Data Explorer. https://gssdataexplorer.norc.org/

15. Taylor, C. A., Hamvas, L., & Paris, R. (2011). Perceived instrumentality and normativeness of corporal punishment use among black mothers. *Family Relations, 60*(1), 60–72.

16. Straus, M. (2009). *Beating the Devil Out of Them: Corporal Punishment in American Families and Its Effects on Children*. New Brunswick, NJ: Transaction.

17. Holden, G. W., Williamson, P. A., & Holland, G. W. O. (2014). Eavesdropping on the family: A pilot investigation of corporal punishment in the home. *Journal of Family Psychology, 28*(3), 401–406. https://doi.org/10.1037/a0036370

18. Bell, T., & Romano, T. (2012). Opinions about child corporal punishment and influencing factors. *Journal of Interpersonal Violence, 27*(11), 2208–2229. https://journals.sagepub.com/doi/10.1177/0886260511432154

19. Holden, G. W., Coleman, S. M., & Schmidt, K. L. (1995). Why 3-year-old children get spanked: Parent and child determinants as reported by college-educated mothers. *Merrill-Palmer Quarterly, 41*(4), 431–452.

20. Lee, S. J., & Altschul, I. (2015). Spanking of young children: Do immigrant and U.S. born Hispanic parents differ? *Journal of Interpersonal Violence, 30*(3), 475–498; MacKenzie, M. J., Nicklas, E., Waldfogel, J., & Brooks-Gunn, J. (2012). Corporal punishment and child behavioural and cognitive outcomes through 5 years of age: Evidence from a *Contemporary Urban Birth Cohort Study*. *Infant and Child Development, 21*, 3–33.

21. Huang, C. C., & Lee, I. (2008). The first three years of parenting: Evidence from the Fragile Families and Child Well Being Study. *Children and Youth Services Review, 30*, 1447–1457; Lee, Y. (2009). Early motherhood and harsh parenting: The role of human, social and cultural capital. *Child Abuse & Neglect, 33*, 625–637.

22. Friedson, M. (2016). Authoritarian parenting attitudes and social origin: The multigenerational relationship of socioeconomic position to childrearing values. *Child Abuse & Neglect, 51*, 263–275.

23. Gage, A. J., & Silvestre, E. A. (2010). Maternal violence, victimization, and child physical punishment in Peru. *Child Abuse & Neglect, 34*, 523–533.

24. Barber, J. S., Axinn, W. G., & Thornton, A. (1999). Unwanted childbearing, health, and mother-child relationships. *Journal of Health and Social Behavior, 40*(3), 231–257.

25. Flynn, C. P. (1994). Regional differences in attitudes toward corporal punishment. *Journal of Marriage and the Family, 56*(2), 314–324.

26. Stolley, K. S., & Szinovacz, M. (1997). Caregiving responsibilities and child spanking. *Journal of Family Violence, 12*(1), 99–112.

27. Gelles, R. J., & Hargreaves, E. F. (1990). Maternal employment and violence toward children. In M. A. Straus & R. J. Gelles (Eds.), *Physical Violence in American Families* (pp. 263–277). New Brunswick, NJ: Transaction.

28. Eamon, M. K. (2001). Antecedents and socioemotional consequences of physical punishment on parents in two-parent families. *Child Abuse & Neglect, 6*, 787–802.

29. Eamon, M. K. (2001). Antecedents and socioemotional consequences of physical punishment on parents in two-parent families. *Child Abuse & Neglect, 6*, 787–802; Knox, M., Rosenberger, R., Sarwar, S., Mangewala, V., & Klag, N. (2015). History of postpartum depression and the odds of maternal corporal punishment. *Family Systems and Health, 33*(4), 395–399.

30. Guzzo, K. B., & Lee, H. (2008). Couple relationship status and patterns in early parenting practices. *Journal of Marriage and the Family, 70*(1), 44–61.

31. Jackson, A. P., Gyamfi, P., Brooks-Gunn, J., & Blake, M. (1988). Employment status, psychological well-being, social support, and physical discipline practices of single black mothers. *Journal of Marriage and the Family, 60*(4), 894–902.

32. Holden, G. W., Miller, P. C., & Harris, S. D. (1999). The instrumental side of corporal punishment: Parents' reported practices and outcome expectancies. *Journal of Marriage and the Family, 61*(4), 908–919.

33. Holden, G. W., Miller, P. C., & Harris, S. D. (1999). The instrumental side of corporal punishment: Parents' reported practices and outcome expectancies. *Journal of Marriage and the Family, 61*(4), 908–919.

34. GSS Data Explorer, NORC. https://gssdataexplorer.norc.org/ g

35. GSS Data Explorer, NORC. https://gssdataexplorer.norc.org/

36. Friedson, M. (2016). Authoritarian parenting attitudes and social origin: The multigenerational relationship of socioeconomic position on childrearing values. *Child Abuse & Neglect, 51*, 263–275. Friedson cites studies that go back to 1969, covering eight different studies confirming this finding.

37. Curtner-Smith, M. E., Bennett, T. L., & O'Rear, M. R. (1995). Father's Occupational Conditions, values of self-direction and conformity, and perceptions of nurturant and restrictive parenting in relation to young children's depression and aggression. *Family Relations, 44*(3), 299–305; Erlanger, H. S. (1974). Social class and corporal punishment in child-rearing: A reassessment. *American Sociological Review, 39*, 68–85; Kohn, M. (1963). Social-class and parent child relationships: An interpretation. *American Journal of Sociology, 68*(4), 471–480; Lareau, A. (2002). Invisible inequality: Social class and child rearing in Black families and White families. *American Sociological Review, 67*(5), 747–776.

38. Lareau, A. (2011). *Unequal Childhoods: Class, Race and Family Life*. Berkeley, CA: University of California Press.

39. Hoff, E., Laursen, B., & Tardif, T. (2002). Socioeconomic status and parenting. In M. H. Bornstein (Ed.), *Handbook of Parenting: Biology and Ecology of Parenting* (Vol. 2, pp. 231–252). Mahwah, NJ: Lawrence Erlbaum Associates; Kohn, M. (1969). *Class and Conformity: A Study in Values*. Homewood, IL: Dorsey Press; Lareau, A. (2011). *Unequal Childhoods: Class, Race and Family Life*. Berkeley, CA: University of California Press; Lipset, S. M. (1959). Democracy and working class authoritarianism. *American Sociological Review, 24*, 482–501; Lipsitz, L. (1965). Working-class authoritarianism, a re-evaluation. *American Sociological Review, 30*, 103–109.

40. Collins, R. (2005). Conflict theory of corporal punishment. In M. Donnelly & M. A. Straus (Eds.), *Corporal Punishment of Children in Theoretical Perspective*. New Haven, CT:. Yale University Press.

41. Bluestone, C., & Tamis-LeMonda, C. S. (1999). Correlates of parenting styles in predominantly working and middle class African-American mothers. *Journal of Marriage and the Family, 61*, 881–893; Conger, R. D., Ge, X., Elder, G. H., Lorenz, F. O., & Simons, R. L. (1994). Economic stress, coercive family process, and developmental problems of adolescents. *Child Development, 65*, 541–561; Giles-Sims, J., Straus, M., & Sugarman, D. (1995). Child, maternal and family characteristics associated with spanking. *Family Relationships, 44*, 170–176; Lipset, S. M. (1959). Democracy and working class authoritarianism. *American Sociological Review, 24*, 482–501; McLoyd, C. (1990). The impact of economic hardship on Black families and children: Psychological distress, parenting, and socioemotional development. *Child Development, 61*, 311–346.

42. Day, R. D., Peterson, G. W., & McCracken, C. (1998). Predicting Spanking of Younger and Older Children by Mothers and Fathers. *Journal of Marriage and Family, 60*(1), 79–94; Giles-Sims, J., Straus, M., & Sugarman, D. (1995). Child, maternal and family characteristics associated with spanking. *Family Relationships, 44*, 170–176; Kohn, M. (1969). *Class and Conformity: A Study in Values*. Homewood, IL: Dorsey Press

43. Friedson, M. (2016). Authoritarian parenting attitudes and social origin: The multigenerational relationship of socioeconomic position on childrearing values. *Child Abuse & Neglect, 51*, 263–275.

44. Anderson, C., & Wimer, C. (2014, March). *The Great Recession and High Frequency Spanking*. Russel Sage Foundation Research Summary. Based on research by Brooks-Gunn, J., Schneider, W., & Waldfogel, J. (2013). The great recession and risk for child maltreatment. *Child Abuse & Neglect, 37*, 721–729..

45. Erlanger, H. S. (1974). Social class and corporal punishment in childrearing: A reassessment. *American Sociological Review, 39*, 68–85.

46. Clement, S. (2015, March 15). Millennials like to spank their kids just as much as their parents did. *The Washington Post*. https://www.washingtonpost.com/news/wonk/wp/2015/03/05/millennials-like-to-spank-their-kids-just-as-much-as-their-parents-did/

47. Zolotor, A. J. (2014). Corporal punishment. *Pediatric Clinics of North America, 61*, 971–978. http://dx.doi.org/10.1016/j.pcl.2014.06.003

48. MacKenzie, M. J., Nicklas, E., Waldfogel, J., & Brooks-Gunn, J. (2012). Corporal punishment and child behavioural and cognitive outcomes through 5 years of age: Evidence from a contemporary urban birth cohort study. *Infant and Child Development, 21*, 3–33.

49. Tang, C. S. (2006). Corporal punishment and physical maltreatment against children: A community study of Chinese parents in Hong Kong. *Child Abuse & Neglect, 30*, 893–907; Murphy-Cowan, T., & Stringer, M. (1999). Physical punishment and the parenting cycle: A survey of Northern Irish parents. *Journal of Community and Applied Social Psychology, 9*, 61–71; Day, R. D., Peterson, G. W., & McCracken, C. (1998). Predicting spanking of younger and older children by mothers and fathers. *Journal of Marriage and the Family, 60*, 79–94.

50. Aikens, N., Tarullo, L., Hulsey, L., Ross, C., West, J., & Xue, Y. (2010). ACF-OPRE report. A year in Head Start: Children, families, and programs. Washington, DC: US Department of Health and Human Services, Administration for Children and Families. https://www.acf.hhs.gov/opre/report/year-head-start-children-families-and-programs

51. Stevens-Long, J. (1973). The effect of behavioral context on some aspects of adult disciplinary practice and affect. *Child Development, 44*, 476–484; Milliones, J. (1978). Relationship between perceived child temperament and maternal behaviors. *Child Development, 49*, 1255–1257; Lee, C. L., & Bates, J. E. (1985). Mother-child interaction at age two years and perceived difficult temperament. *Child Development, 45*, 1314–1325; Gordon, B. N. (1983). Maternal perception of child temperament and observed mother-child interaction. *Child Psychiatry and Human Development, 13*, 153–166; Eisenberg, N., & Fabes, R. A. (1994). Mothers' reactions to children's negative emotions: Relations to children's temperament and anger behavior. *Merrill-Palmer Quarterly, 40*, 138–156; Day, R. D., Peterson, G. W., & McCracken, C. (1998). Predicting spanking of younger and older children by mothers and fathers. *Journal of Marriage and the Family, 60*(1), 79.

52. Combes-Orme, T., & Cain, D. S. (2008). Predictors of mother's use of spanking with their infants. *Child Abuse & Neglect, 32*, 649–657; Mackenzie, M. J., Nicklas, E., Brooks-Gunn, J., & Waldfogel, J. (2011). Who spanks infants and toddlers? Evidence from the Fragile Families and Child Well-Being Study. *Children and Youth Services Review, 33*, 1364–1373.

53. Regalado, M., Sareen, H., Inkelas, M., Wissow, L. S., & Halfon, N. (2004). Parents' discipline of young children: Results from the National Survey on Early Childhood Health. *Pediatrics, 113*(6), 1952–1958.

54. MacKenzie, M. J., Nicklas, E., Waldfogel, J., & Brooks-Gunn, J. (2012). Corporal punishment and child behavioural and cognitive outcomes through 5 years of age: Evidence from a contemporary urban birth cohort study. *Infant and Child Development, 21*, 3–33.

55. Clifford, E. (1959). Discipline in the home: A controlled observational study of parental practices. *Journal of Genetic Psychology, 95*, 45–82; Holden, G. W., Coleman, S. M., & Schmidt, K. L. (1995). Why 3-year-old children get spanked: Parent and child determinants as reported by college-educated mothers. *Merrill-Palmer Quarterly, 41*(4), 431–452.

56. Regalado, M., Sareen, H., Inkelas, M., Wissow, L. S., & Halfon, N. (2004). Parents' discipline of young children: Results from the National Survey on Early Childhood Health. *Pediatrics, 113*(6), 1952–1958.

57. MacKenzie, M. J., Nicklas, E., Waldfogel, J., & Brooks-Gunn, J. (2012). Corporal punishment and child behavioural and cognitive outcomes through 5 years of age: Evidence from a contemporary urban birth cohort study. *Infant and Child Development, 21*, 3–33.

58. Becker, W. C. (1964). Consequences of different models of parental discipline. In M. L. Hoffman & W. L. Hoffman (Eds.), *Review of Child Development Research.* (Vol. 1, pp. 169–208). New York: Sage.

59. Straus, M. (1994). *Beating the Devil Out of Them: Corporal Punishment in American Families and Its Effects on Children.* New York: Lexington Books.

60. Gunnoe, M. L., & Mariner, C. L. (1997). Toward a developmental-contextual model of the effects of parental spanking on children's aggression. *Archives of Pediatrics and Adolescent Medicine, 151*, 768–775.

61. O'Kane, C. (2018, September 11). Georgia school reinstating paddling to punish students. *CBS News.* https://www.cbsnews.com/news/georgia-school-reinstating-paddling-to-punish-students/

Chapter 2

1. DeMause, L. (1974). *The History of Childhood* (p. 51). Lanham, MD: Rowman & Littlefield.

2. Aries, P. (1965). *Centuries of Childhood: A Social History of Family Life.* New York: Knopf Doubleday.

3. Pinker, D. (2012). *The Better Angels of Our Nature: Why Violence Has Declined.* New York: Penguin; Kempe C. H., & Helfer, R. E. (1980). *The Battered Child Syndrome* (3rd ed.). Chicago: University of Chicago Press.

4. Radbill, S. X., Kempe, C. H., & Helfer, R. E. (1968). *A History of Child Abuse and Infanticide.* Chicago: University of Chicago Press.

5. *End Violence Against Children.* Retrieved September 2021. States Committed to Law Reform. https://endcorporalpunishment.org/committed-states/

6. DeMause, L. (1974). *The History of Childhood* (p. 164). Lanham, MD: Rowman & Littlefield.

7. DeMause, L. (1974). *The History of Childhood* (p. 1). Lanham, MD: Rowman & Littlefield.

8. Pinker, D. (2012). *The Better Angels of Our Nature: Why Violence Has Declined.* New York: Penguin.

9. Davis, P. W., Chandler, J. L., & LaRossa, R. (2004). "I've tried the switch but he laughs through the tears:" The use and conceptualization of corporal punishment during the Machine Age, 1924–1939. *Child Abuse and Neglect, 28,* 1291–1310.

10. Earle, A. M. (1993). *Child Life in Colonial Days.* Massachusetts: Berkshire House.

11. Sidman, L. R. (1972). The Massachusetts Stubborn Child Law: Law and order in the home. *Family Law Quarterly, 1,* 33–58.

12. Sutton, J. R. (1981). Stubborn children: Law and the socialization of deviance in the Puritan colonies. *Family Law Quarterly, 1,* 3–64.

13. Donnelly, M. (2005). Putting corporal punishment of children in historical perspective In M. Donnelly & M. A. Straus (Eds.), *Corporal Punishment of Children in Theoretical Perspective* (pp. 41–54). New Haven, CT: Yale University Press.

14. Miller, A. (1983). *For Your Own Good* (p. 13). New York: Farrar, Straus, Giroux. Miller cites J. Sulzer from 1748.

15. Locke, J. *Some Thoughts Concerning Education.* Hoboken, NJ: Generic NL Freebook. Citation taken from Gathorne-Hardy, J. (1972). *The Unnatural History of the Nanny* (p. 52). New York: The Dial Press.

16. Gathorne-Hardy, J. (1972). *The Unnatural History of the Nanny.* New York: The Dial Press.

17. Miller, D. R., & Swanson G. E. (1958). *The Changing American Parent* (p. 8). New York: John Wiley and Sons.

18. Pinker, D. (2012). *The Better Angels of Our Nature: Why Violence Has Declined.* New York: Penguin.

19. Cable, M. (1975). *The Little Darlings: A History of American Children* (p. 76). New York: Charles Scribner's Sons.

20. Cable, M. (1975). *The Little Darlings: A History of American Children* (pp. 74–77). New York: Charles Scribner's Sons. The author cites a book published in 1830 titled, *An Astonishing Affair,* by the minister who whipped the child.

21. Cobb, L. (1847). *Evil Tendencies of Corporal Punishment as a Mean of Moral Discipline in Families and Schools, Examined and Discussed.* New York: Mark H. Newman & Co.

22. Miller, D. R., & Swanson, G. E. (1958). *The Changing American Parent* (p. 7). New York: John Wiley and Sons.

23. Cable, M. (1975). *The Little Darlings: A History of American Children.* New York: Charles Scribner's Sons.

24. Miller, D. R., & Swanson, G. E. (1958). *The Changing American Parent* (p. 212). New York: John Wiley and Sons.

25. Miller, D. R., & Swanson, G. E. (1958). *The Changing American Parent*. New York: John Wiley and Sons.

26. Donnelly, M. (2005). *Putting Corporal Punishment of Children in Historical Perspective*. In M. Donnelly & M. A. Straus (Eds.), *Corporal Punishment of Children in Theoretical Perspective* (pp. 41–54). Yale University Press: New Haven.

27. Belle, M. (1884, June). Hasty mothers. *Ladies Home Journal*, as described in Miller, D. R., & Swanson G. E. (1958). *The Changing American Parent*. New York: John Wiley and Sons.

28. Miller D. R., & Swanson, G. E. (1958). *The Changing American Parent* (p. 13). New York: John Wiley and Sons.

29. Gordon, L. (1988). *Heroes of Their Own Lives: The Politics and History of Family Violence*. New York: Viking Penguin.

30. Gordon, L. (1988). *Heroes of Their Own Lives: The Politics and History of Family Violence* (p.179). New York: Viking Penguin.

31. McNally, R. B. (1981). *Nearly a Century Later—The Child Savers—Child Advocates and the Juvenile Justice System*. National Institute of Justice. https://www.ncjrs.gov/App/Publicati ons/abstract.aspx?ID=80064

32. Miller, D. R., & Swanson, G. E. (1958). *The Changing American Parent* (p. 9). New York: John Wiley and Sons.

33. Raw, N. (1929). Royal Medico-Psychological Association Annual Meeting: Fear. *Lancet*, August, 254.

34. Quilliard, M. J. (1928). *Child Study Discussion Records* (p. 16). Property of the Child Study Association. Social Welfare History Archives., University of Minnesota Libraries.

35. Quilliard, M. J. (1928). *Child Study Discussion Records* (p. 19). Property of the Child Study Association. Social Welfare History Archives, University of Minnesota Libraries.

36. Child Study Association of America, North Harlem, New York Branch, Papers from 1930–1933. Summary of Questionnaires filled out by Members, 1932. Social Welfare History Archives, University of Minnesota Libraries.

37. Hopkirk, H. (1929). *Are Children's Institutions Obsolete?* Papers, articles, and speeches. (Box 1). Social Welfare History Archives, University of Minnesota Libraries.

38. Park, A. (1930, June 30). Stop whipping children. *Journal of Education, 111*(22), 626–627.

39. Park, A. (1930, June 30). Stop whipping children. *Journal of Education, 111*(22), 626–627.

40. Barry, E. S. (1926). Minutes and papers from the Child Study Association of America Study Groups, Chapter 128. Social Welfare History Archives, University of Minnesota Libraries.

41. Myers, G. C. (1938, May). Classroom clinic of personality and behavior problems. *Journal of Education, 121*(5), 168–169.

42. Zelizer, V. A. (1985). *Pricing the Priceless Child: The Changing Social Value of Children*. New York: Basic Books.

43. Patri, A. (1948). *How to Help Your Child Grow Up: Suggestions for Guiding Children From Birth Through Adolescence*. New York: Rand McNally & Company.

44. Angelo Patri papers, Library of Congress. 1904–1962 (bulk 1924–1962). https://lccn.loc. gov/mm74047167, and newspaper articles in *Chronicling America: Historic American Newspapers* https://chroniclingamerica.loc.gov/. Also: Patri, A. (1940). *The Parents Daily Counselor*. New York: The Wise Parlow Company; Patri, A. (1948). *How to Help Your Child Grow Up: Suggestions for Guiding Children From Birth Through Adolescence*. Chicago: Rand McNally. Patri (September 30, 1938).

45. Angelo Patri papers, Library of Congress. 1904–1962 (March 11, 1936). https://lccn.loc.gov/mm74047167, and newspaper articles in *Chronicling America: Historic American Newspapers* https://chroniclingamerica.loc.gov/.

46. Angelo Patri papers, Library of Congress. 1904–1962. (March 29, 1931) https://lccn.loc.gov/mm74047167, and newspaper articles in *Chronicling America: Historic American Newspapers* https://chroniclingamerica.loc.gov/. .

47. Angelo Patri papers, Library of Congress. 1904–1962. (May 1, 1938) https://lccn.loc.gov/mm74047167, and newspaper articles in *Chronicling America: Historic American Newspapers* https://chroniclingamerica.loc.gov/. .

48. Freiberg, S. (1959). *The Magic Years* (pp. 253–254). New York: Charles Scribner's Sons.

49. O'Neil, M. (1952). Spank him or soothe him? Life and Health. *National Health Journal, 67*(3), 12–15.

50. Simpson, R. H. (1942, March). A basic approach to remedial reading. *English Journal, 31*(3), 219–226.

51. Dreikurs, R., & Soltz, V. (1964). *Children: The Challenge* (pp. 68–69). New York: Meredith Press.

52. Dreikurs, R., & Soltz, V. (1964). *Children: The Challenge* (pp. 76–77). New York: Meredith Press.

53. Edelman, P. (1977). Nationwide Drive of Children's Rights. In Gross, B., & Gross, R. *The Children's Rights Movement: Overcoming the Oppression of Young People.* New York: Anchor Press/Doubleday.

54. Krumboltz, J. D. (1972*). Changing Children's Behavior* (p. 206). Englewood Cliffs, NJ: Prentice-Hall.

55. Dodson, F. (1970). *How to Parent* (p. 7). Secaucus, NJ: Castle Books.

56. Dreikurs, R., & Grey, L. (1970). *A Parents' Guide to Child Discipline* (p. 32). New York: Hawthorne.

57. CAN Week. (1982). Rod McKuen's itinerary. Script read for a week of proclamation in the city of New York. National Committee for the Prevention of Child Abuse (Box 31). Social Welfare History Archives, University of Minnesota Libraries.

58. Krumboltz, J. D. (1972). *Changing Children's Behavior* (p. 190). Englewood Cliffs, NJ: Prentice-Hall.

59. Miller, A. (1983). *For Your Own Good: Hidden Cruelty in Child Rearing and the Roots of Violence.* New York: Farrar, Straus, Giroux.

60. Miller, A. (1983). *For Your Own Good: Hidden Cruelty in Child Rearing and the Roots of Violence* (p. 64). New York: Farrar, Straus, Giroux.

61. Miller, A. (1990). *Banished Knowledge: Facing Childhood Injuries.* New York: Doubleday.

62. Samalin, N. (1987). *Loving Your Child Is Not Enough: Positive Discipline That Works.* New York: Viking.

63. Reisser, P. C. (1994). *Complete Book of Baby and Child Care* (p. 307). Wheaton, IL: Tyndale.

64. Samalin, N. (1991). *Love and Anger: The Parental Dilemma* (p. 60). New York: Penguin Books.

65. Straus, M. (1994). *Beating the Devil Out of Them: Corporal Punishment in American Families and Its Effect on Children.* San Francisco: Jossey-Bass/Lexington.

66. Straus, M. (1994). *Beating the Devil Out of Them: Corporal Punishment in American Families and Its Effect on Children.* San Francisco: Jossey-Bass/Lexington.

67. Frost, J. (2014). *Toddler Rules: Your 5 Step Guide for Shaping Proper Behavior.* New York: Ballantine.

68. Greven, P. J. (1990). *Spare the Child: The Religious Roots of Punishment and the Psychological Impact of Physical Abuse*. New York: Vintage Books.

69. Greven, P. J. (1990). *Spare the Child: The Religious Roots of Punishment and the Psychological Impact of Physical Abuse* (pp. 48–49). New York: Vintage Books.

70. Greven, P. J. (1990). *Spare the Child: The Religious Roots of Punishment and the Psychological Impact of Physical Abuse*. New York: Vintage Books.

71. Greven, P. J. (1990). *Spare the Child: The Religious Roots of Punishment and the Psychological Impact of Physical Abuse*. New York: Vintage Books.

72. Tomczak, L. (1982). *God, The Rod and Your Child's Bod: The Art of Loving Correction for Christian Parents*. Old Tappan, NJ: Power Books.

73. Greven, P. J. (1990). *Spare the Child: The Religious Roots of Punishment and the Psychological Impact of Physical Abuse*. New York: Vintage Books.

74. Patton, S. (2017). *Spare the Kids: Why Whupping Children Won't Save Black America*. Boston: Beacon Press. Her commentary on the transformation of beatings to spankings for White children but not children of color is also based on Fleck, E. (1987). *Domestic Tyranny: The Making of American Social Policy Against Family Violence From Colonial Times to Present*. New York: Oxford University Press.

75. Dr. Alvin Pouissant, as quoted in Patton, S. (2017). *Spare the Kids: Why Whupping Children Won't Save Black America* (p. 141). Boston: Beacon Press.

76. Greven, P. J. (1990). *Spare the Child: The Religious Roots of Punishment and the Psychological Impact of Physical Abuse*. New York: Vintage Books.

77. Churches Network for NonViolence, Global Initiative to End all Corporal Punishment of Children and Save the Children. (2015). *Ending Corporal Punishment of Children: A Handbook for Working With Religious Communities*.

78. Greven, P. J. (1990). *Spare the Child: The Religious Roots of Punishment and the Psychological Impact of Physical Abuse*. (pp. 100–101). New York: Vintage Books.

79. Coontz, S. (1997). *The Way We Really Are: Coming to Terms With America's Changing Families*. New York: Basic Books.

Chapter 3

1. Moffatt, G. K. (2002). *Violent Heart: Understanding Aggressive Individuals* (p. viii). Westport, CT: Praeger.

2. Allen, A., & Morton, A. (1961). *This Is Your Child: The Story of the National Society for the Prevention of Cruelty to Children*. London: Routledge.

3. Helfer, R. E., & Kempe, C. H. (Eds.). (1968). *The Battered Child*. Chicago: University of Chicago Press.

4. The New York Society for the Prevention of Cruelty to Children. (2000). 125th Anniversary 1875–2000.

5. Ten Bensel, R. W., Rheinberger, M. M., & Radbill, S. X. (1997). Children in a world of violence: The roots of child maltreatment. M. E. Helfer, R. S. Kempe, & R. D. Krugman (Eds.). (1997). *The Battered Child* (5th ed.). Chicago: University of Chicago Press.

6. Helfer, R. E., & Kempe, C. H. (Eds.). (1968). *The Battered Child*. Chicago: University of Chicago Press.

7. Gordon, L. (1988). *Heroes of Their Own Lives: The Politics and History of Family Violence*. New York: Viking Press.

8. Korbin, J. E., & Krugman, R. D. (2015). *Child Maltreatment: Contemporary Issues in Research and Policy*. New York: Springer.

9. Gordon, L. (1988). *Heroes of Their Own Lives: The Politics and History of Family Violence*. New York: Viking Penguin.

10. Helfer, M. E., Kempe, R. S., & Krugman, R. D. (Eds.). (1997). *The Battered Child* (5th ed.). Chicago: University of Chicago Press.

11. Helfer, R. E., & Kempe, C. H. (Eds.). (1968). *The Battered Child*. Chicago: University of Chicago Press.

12. Krugman, R. D., Korbin, J. E., & Kempe, C. H. (2013). *C. Henry Kempe: A 50 Year Legacy to the Field of Child Abuse and Neglect*. New York: Springer.

13. Helfer, R. E., & Kempe, C. H. (Eds.). (1968). *The Battered Child*. Chicago: University of Chicago Press.

14. Helfer, R. E., & Kempe, C. H. (Eds.). (1968). *The Battered Child*. Chicago: University of Chicago Press.

15. Helfer, R. E., & Kempe, C. H. (Eds.). (1968). *The Battered Child*. Chicago: University of Chicago Press.

16. Helfer, R. E., & Kempe, C. H. (Eds.). (1968). *The Battered Child*. Chicago: University of Chicago Press.

17. Helfer, R. E., & Kempe, C. H. (Eds.). (1968). *The Battered Child*. Chicago: University of Chicago Press.

18. NewsWest9. (2016, May 20). *Odessa father strikes child missing goal*. Odessa, Texas. https://www.newswest9.com/article/news/local/police-odessa-father-strikes-child-for-missing-goal/513-00121ef7-169c-4bf1-9cfa-c07d3a95e830

19. Illinois Department of Children and Family Services. (1982). *Child Abuse and Neglect Investigation Decisions Handbook*. Social Welfare History Archives, University of Minnesota Libraries.

20. Lally, J. R., Lerner, C., & E. Lurie-Hurvitz, E. (2001). National survey reveals gaps in the public's and parents' knowledge about early childhood development. *Young Children, 56*(2), 49–53. National Association for the Education of Young Children (NAEYC).

21. Gordon, L. (1988). *Heroes of Their Own Lives: The Politics and History of Family Violence*. New York: Viking.

22. Helfer, R. E., & Kempe, C. H. (Eds.). (1968). *The Battered Child* (pp. 109–110). Chicago: University of Chicago Press.

23. Helfer, R. E., & Kempe, C. H. (Eds.). (1968). *The Battered Child* (p. 106). Chicago: University of Chicago Press.

24. Helfer, R. E., & Kempe, C. H. (Eds.). (1968). *The Battered Child* (p. 104). Chicago: University of Chicago Press.

25. National Committee for the Prevention of Child Abuse. (1984). *Beyond 1984: The Exciting History and Brave New Future of the National Committee for Prevention of Child Abuse* (p. 1). Booklet. National Social Welfare History Archives, University of Minnesota Libraries.

26. The Museum of Classic Chicago Television, Public Service Announcement, Prevent Child Abuse—"Stressed Mom." https://www.youtube.com/wath?v=zCUQY2v5meg

27. Campbell-Ewald Company Research Department. (1985). A comprehension and re-action study of the National Committee for the Prevention of Child Abuse's "Take Time Out" Commercial (Box 29). National Committee for the Prevention of Child Abuse. Social Welfare History Archives, University of Minnesota Libraries.

28. Homan Cook, J. (1976). *Trainee Manual, Focus. Child Abuse and Neglect: Interventions for Social Welfare/Public Health Nursing Providers* (p. 23). Oakland, CA: Children's Trauma Center, Social Welfare History Archives, University of Minnesota Libraries.

29. Homan Cook, J. (1976). *Trainee Manual, Focus. Child Abuse and Neglect: Interventions for Social Welfare/Public Health Nursing Providers* (p. 23). Oakland, CA: Children's Trauma Center, Social Welfare History Archives, University of Minnesota Libraries.

30. National Committee for the Prevention of Child Abuse. (1983). Proposal to the US Federal Government titled, "Determining How a National Public Awareness Campaign Can Help Prevent Child Abuse" (Box 29). Social Welfare History Archives, University of Minnesota Libraries.

31. Coolsen, P. (1981). *Community Involvement in the Prevention of Child Abuse and Neglect.* Third International Congress on Child Abuse and Neglect. National Committee for the Prevention of Child Abuse (Box 30). Social Welfare History Archives, University of Minnesota Libraries.

32. Martinez, E. CBS News affiliate, WKMG. (2011, March 4). *Fla boy, 3, beaten to death for wetting his pants say cops.* Orlando, FL. https://www.cbsnews.com/news/fla-boy-3-beaten-to-death-for-wetting-his-pants-say-cops/

33. Reid, B. V., & Valsiner, J. (1986). Consistency, praise and love: Folk theories of American parents. *Ethos, 14*(3), 282–304.

34. Hazel, N., Ghate, D., Creighton, S., Field, J., & Finch, S. (2003). Violence against children: Threshold of acceptance for physical punishment in a normative study of parents, children and discipline (p. 60). In E. Stanko (Ed.), *The Meanings of Violence.* London: Routledge.

35. Radl, S. L. (1980). American baby: To spank or not to spank. *American Association for Maternal and Child Health, 42, 42.*

36. Hazel, N., Ghate, D. Creighton, S., Field, J., & Finch, S. (2003). Violence against children: Threshold of acceptance for physical punishment in a normative study of parents, children and discipline. In E. Stanko (Ed.), *The Meanings of Violence* (p. 60). London: Routledge.

37. Gonzalez, M., Durrant, J. E., Chabot, M., Trocmé, N., & Brown, J. (2008). What predicts injury from physical punishment? A test of the typologies of violence hypothesis. *Child Abuse and Neglect, 32,* 752–765.

38. Durrant, J. (2002). Distinguishing physical punishment from physical abuse: Implications for professionals. *Canada's Children, 9,* 17–21.

39. Whipple, E. E., & Richey, C. A. (1997). Crossing the line from physical discipline to child abuse: How much is too much? *Child Abuse and Neglect, 21*(5), 431–444.; Fréchette, A., Zoratti, M., & Romano, E. (2015). What is the link between corporal punishment and child physical abuse? *Journal of Family Violence 30,* 135–148.

40. Zolotor, A. J., Theodore, A. D., Chang, J. J., Berjoff, M. C., & Runyan, D. K. (2008). Speak softly and forget the stick: Corporal punishment and child physical abuse. *American Journal of Preventive Medicine, 35,* 364–369.

41. Lee, S. J., Grogan-Kaylor, A., & Berger, L. M. (2014). Parental spanking of 1-year-old children and subsequent child protective services involvement. *Child Abuse and Neglect, 38,* 875–883.

42. Helfer, R. E., & Kempe, C. H. (Eds.). (1968). *The Battered Child* (p. 104). Chicago: The University of Chicago Press.

43. Hazel, N., Ghate, D., Creighton, S., Field, J., & Finch, S. (2003). Violence against children: Threshold of acceptance for physical punishment in a normative study of parents, children and discipline. In E. Stanko (Ed.), *The Meanings of Violence*. London: Routledge.

44. US Department of Health and Human Services, Administration for Children and Families, Administration on Children, Youth and Families, Children's Bureau. (2020). *Child Maltreatment 2018.* https://www.acf.hhs.gov/cb/research-data-technology/statistics-research/child-maltreatment

45. Dwyer, J. G. (2010). Parental entitlement and corporal punishment. *Law and Contemporary Problems, 73*(2), 189–210.

46. Dwyer, J. G. (2010). Parental entitlement and corporal punishment. *Law and Contemporary Problems, 73*(2), 189–210.

47. Davis, P. W. (2003). *Social Problems Constructionist Readings*. Hawthorne, NY: Aldine de Gruyter.

48. US Department of Health and Human Services, Administration for Children and Families, Administration on Children, Youth and Families, Children's Bureau. (2020). *Child Maltreatment 2018.*https://www.acf.hhs.gov/cb/research-data-technology/statistics-research/child-maltreatment

49. Child Welfare Information Gateway. (2019). *Definitions of child abuse and neglect*. Washington, DC: US Department of Health and Human Services, Children's Bureau.

50. Cope, K. C. (2010). The age of discipline: The relevance of age to the reasonableness of corporal punishment. *Law and Contemporary Problems, 73*(2), 167–188.

51. All Things Considered. (2007, February 1). Move to criminalize spanking sparks questions. Opposing viewpoints in context. http://link.galegroup.com/apps/doc/A158699645/OVIC?u=clic_augsburg&sid=OVIC&xid=5d00c61e; Sanders, J. (2007, January 19). Measure seeks to punish spanking: Bill would make state first to ban swatting of children under 4. *The Sacramento Bee.*

52. ABCNEWS.com. (2007, November 28). Massachusetts could become first state to outlaw corporal punishment. http://abcnews.go.com/WN/story?id=3921895

53. Gordon, L. (1988). *Heroes of Their Own Lives: The Politics and History of Family Violence*. New York: Viking Penguin.

54. Lee, S. J., Grogan-Kaylor, A., & Berger, L. M. (2014). Parental spanking of 1-year-old children and subsequent child protective services involvement. *Child Abuse and Neglect, 38*(5), 875–883; Taylor, C. A., Guterman, N. B., Lee, S. J., & Rathouz, P. J. (2009). Intimate partner violence, maternal stress, nativity, and risk for maternal maltreatment of young children. *American Journal of Public Health, 99*(1), 175–183. http://dx.doi.org/10.2105/AJPH.2007.126722

55. Korbin, J. E., & Krugman, R. D. (2015). *Child Maltreatment: Contemporary Issues in Research and Policy* (p. xxiv). New York: Springer.

56. US Department of Health and Human Services, Administration for Children and Families, Administration on Children, Youth and Families, Children's Bureau. (2019). *Child Maltreatment 2017.* https://www.acf.hhs.gov/cb/research-data-technology/statistics-research/child-maltreatment

57. Child Welfare Information Gateway. (2019). *Child maltreatment 2017: Summary of key findings*. Washington, DC: US Department of Health and Human Services, Administration for Children and Families, Children's Bureau. https://www.childwelfare.gov/pubs/factsheets/canstats/

58. Child Welfare Information Gateway. (2019). *Child maltreatment 2017: Summary of key findings*. Washington, DC: US Department of Health and Human Services, Administration for Children and Families, Children's Bureau. https://www.childwelfare.gov/pubs/factshe ets/canstats/

59. Illinois Department of Children and Family Services. (1982). *Child Abuse and Neglect Investigation Decisions Handbook*. Social Welfare History Archives, University of Minnesota Libraries.

60. Illinois Department of Children and Family Services. (1982). *Child Abuse and Neglect Investigation Decisions Handbook* (p. 112). Social Welfare History Archives, University of Minnesota Libraries.

61. Ho, G. W. K., & Gross, D. A. (2015). Differentiating physical discipline from abuse: Findings from Chinese American mothers and pediatric nurses. *Child Abuse and Neglect, 43*, 83–94.

62. Helfer, M. E., Kempe, R. S., & Krugman, R. D. (Eds.). (1997). *The Battered Child* (5th ed., p. 61). Chicago: The University of Chicago Press.

63. Gilligan, J. (2000). Punishment and violence: Is the criminal law based on one huge mistake? *Social Research, 67*, 745–773. Gilligan describes a process outlined by Scheff, T., & Retizinger, S. M. (1991). *Emotions and Violence: Shame and Rage in Destructive Conflicts*. New York: Lexington Books.

64. Davies, P. W. (1999). Corporal punishment cessation: Social contexts and parents experiences. *Journal of Interpersonal Violence, 14*(5), 498.

65. Radl, S. L. (1980). American baby: To spank or not to spank. *American Association for Maternal and Child Health, 42*, 42.

66. Gagné, M., Tourigny, M., Joly, J., & Pouliot-Lapointe, J. (2007). Predictors of adult attitudes toward corporal punishment of children. *Journal of Interpersonal Violence, 22*(10), 1285–1304.

67. Ramirez, J. (2018). *Jolly K.'s Courageous Contribution*. Surf Net Parents, https://www.sur fnetparents.com/4882/jolly-k-s-courageous-contribution/; Raz, M. (2017). Lessons From History: Parents Anonymous and Child Abuse Prevention Policy. *Pediatrics, 140*(6). https:// doi.org/10.1542/peds.2017-0340, *Courier-News*. (1980, November 21). Bridgewater, NJ p. 20; Rafael, T., & Pion-Berlin, L. (1999, April). *Juvenile justice bulletin*. US Department of Justice Office of Justice Programs Office of Juvenile Justice and Delinquency Prevention. ; Nelson, B. J. (2016). *Making an Issue of Child Abuse*. Chicago: University of Chicago Press.

68. Rafael, T., & Pion-Berlin, L. (1999, April). *Juvenile justice bulletin* (p. 2). US Department of Justice Office of Justice Programs Office of Juvenile Justice and Delinquency Prevention.

69. Rafael, T., & Pion-Berlin, L. (1999, April). *Juvenile justice bulletin* (p. 6). US Department of Justice Office of Justice Programs Office of Juvenile Justice and Delinquency Prevention.

70. Ramirez, J. (2018). *Jolly K.'s Courageous Contribution*. Surf Net Parents. https://www.surfnet parents.com/4882/jolly-k-s-courageous-contribution/

71. Wilkins, N., Myers, L., Kuehl., T., Bauman, A., & Hertz, M. (2018). Connecting the dots: State health department approaches to addressing shared risk and protective factors across multiple forms of violence. *Journal of Public Health Management Practice, 24*(Suppl. 1), 32–41.

72. Wilkins, N., Myers, L., Kuehl., T., Bauman, A., & Hertz, M. (2018). Connecting the dots: State health department approaches to addressing shared risk and protective factors across multiple forms of violence. *Journal of Public Health Management Practice, 24*(Suppl. 1), 32–41.

73. Wilkins, N., Myers, L., Kuehl., T., Bauman, A., & Hertz, M. (2018). Connecting the dots: State health department approaches to addressing shared risk and protective factors across multiple forms of violence. *Journal of Public Health Management Practice, 24*(Suppl. 1), 32–41.

74. Wilkins, N., Myers, L., Kuehl., T., Bauman, A., & Hertz, M. (2018). Connecting the dots: State health department approaches to addressing shared risk and protective factors across multiple forms of violence. *Journal of Public Health Management Practice, 24*(Suppl. 1), 32–41.

75. Gilligan, J. (2001). *Preventing Violence*. New York: Thames & Hudson.

76. Korbin, J. E., & Krugman, R. D. (2015). *Child Maltreatment: Contemporary Issues in Research and Policy* (p. 230). New York: Springer.

77. Most states ban physical punishment by foster parents. Confirmation lies in individual state statute. Many of these can be found at the National Center for Child Welfare at the Silberman School of Social Work (http://www.nccwe.org/index.html) and Embrella, Embracing and Empowering Families. (2016). *Positive Discipline: How to Discipline Your Foster Child*. http://foster-adoptive-kinship-family-services-nj.org/discipline-your-foster-child/

Chapter 4

1. Hooper, C., & Woodruff, C. S. (1928, April 30). The journal mailbag: This unspanked generation. *Journal of Education, 107*(18), 542–543.

2. Pearl, M., & Pearl, D. (1994). *To Train Up a Child*. Pleasantville TN: No Greater Joy Ministries.

3. Pearl, M., & Pearl, D. (1994). *To Train Up a Child* (p. 40). Pleasantville, TN: No Greater Joy Ministries.

4. Straus, M. A. (2008). Bucking the tide in family violence research. *Trauma, Violence, & Abuse, 9*,(4), 191–213.

5. Dobson, J. (1992). *The New Dare to Discipline* (p. 22). Wheaton, IL: Tyndale Press.

6. Straus, M. A. (2008). Bucking the tide in family violence research. *Trauma, Violence, & Abuse, 9*(4), 191–213.

7. Martin, D. (1976). *Battered Wives*. San Francisco: Glide; and Langley, R., & Levy, R. C. (1977). *Wife Beating: The Silent Crisis*. New York: E. P. Dutton.

8. Straus, M. (1994). *Beating the Devil Out of Them: Corporal Punishment in American Families and Its Effect on Children* (p. 4). San Francisco: Jossey-Bass/Lexington.

9. Straus, M. (1994). *Beating the Devil Out of Them: Corporal Punishment in American Families and its Effect on Children* (p. 4). San Francisco: Jossey-Bass/Lexington.

10. Steinmetz, S. K., & Straus, M. A.(1973). Family as the cradle of violence. *Society, 10*(6), 50–56.

11. Straus, M. (1994). *Beating the Devil Out of Them: Corporal Punishment in American Families and its Effect on Children* (p. 19). San Francisco: Jossey-Bass/Lexington.

12. Obituary of Dr. Murray Straus. https://www.legacy.com/obituaries/unionleader/obituary.aspx?page=lifestory&pid=180009152

13. Straus, M. (1994). *Beating the Devil Out of Them: Corporal Punishment in American Families and its Effect on Children* (pp. ii–iii). San Francisco: Jossey-Bass/Lexington.

14. Straus, M. A. (2008). Bucking the tide in family violence research (p. 196). *Trauma, Violence, & Abuse, 9*(4), 191–213.
15. Straus, M. A. (2008). Bucking the tide in family violence research (p. 191). *Trauma, Violence, & Abuse, 9*(4), 191–213.
16. Finkelhor, D. (2017). Straus dedication. *Child Abuse and Neglect,* 1–2.
17. Dobson, J. (1970). *Dare to Discipline: A Psychologist Offers Urgent Advice to Parents and Teachers.* Wheaton, IL: Tyndale House Publishers.
18. Dobson, J. (1970). *Dare to Discipline: A Psychologist Offers Urgent Advice to Parents and Teachers.* Wheaton, IL: Tyndale House Publishers.
19. Dobson, J. (1970). *Dare to Discipline: A Psychologist Offers Urgent Advice to Parents and Teachers* (p. 28). Wheaton, IL: Tyndale House Publishers.
20. Dobson, J. (1970). *Dare to Discipline: A Psychologist Offers Urgent Advice to Parents and Teachers.* Wheaton, IL: Tyndale House Publishers.
21. Dobson, J. (1970). *Dare to Discipline: A Psychologist Offers Urgent Advice to Parents and Teachers.* Wheaton, IL: Tyndale House Publishers.
22. Dobson, J. (1970). *Dare to Discipline: A Psychologist Offers Urgent Advice to Parents and Teachers* (p. 24). Wheaton, IL: Tyndale House Publishers.
23. Dobson, J. (1970). *Dare to Discipline: A Psychologist Offers Urgent Advice to Parents and Teachers.* Wheaton, IL: Tyndale House Publishers.
24. Dobson, J. (1970). *Dare to Discipline: A Psychologist Offers Urgent Advice to Parents and Teachers* (p. 30). Wheaton, IL: Tyndale House Publishers.
25. James Dobson, PhD. https://www.focusonthefamily.com/contributors/james-dobson-ph-d/
26. Gladwell, M. (2002). *The Tipping Point: How Little Things Can Make a Big Difference.* New York: Little, Brown.
27. Dobson, J. (1992). *The New Dare to Discipline* (p. 12). Wheaton, IL: Tyndale Press.
28. Dobson, J. (1992). *The New Dare to Discipline* (p. 35). Wheaton, IL: Tyndale Press.
29. Dr. James Dobson's blog. https://www.drjamesdobson.org/blogs/dr-dobson-blog/dr-dobson-blog/2015/11/09/5-reasons-why-spanking-fails
30. Dobson, J. (1992). *The New Dare to Discipline.* Wheaton, IL: Tyndale Press.
31. Comer, J. P., & Poussaint, A. F. (1975). *Black Child Care.* New York: Simon & Schuster.
32. Comer, J. P., & Poussaint, A. F. (1975). *Black Child Care* (p. 57). New York: Simon & Schuster
33. Comer, J. P., & Poussaint, A. F. (1992). *Raising Black Children* (p. 49). New York: Penguin.
34. Comer, J. P., & Poussaint, A. F. (1975). *Black Child Care* (p. 55). New York: Simon & Schuster.
35. Comer, J. P., & Poussaint, A. F. (1992). *Raising Black Children* (p. 51). New York: Penguin.
36. Heilmann, A., Mehay A., Watt, R. G., Kelly, Y., Durrant, J. E., van Turnhout, J., & Gershoff, E. T. (2021). Physical punishment and child outcomes: A narrative review of prospective studies. *Lancet, 398,* 355–364. https://doi.org/10.1016/S0140-6736(21)00582-1; Grogan-Kaylor, A., Ma, J., & Graham-Bermann, S. A. (2009). The case against physical punishment. *Current Opinion in Psychology, 19,* 22–27.
37. Sears, R. R., Maccoby, E. C., & Levin, H. (1957). *Patterns of Childrearing.* New York: Row, Peterson.
38. Burt, S. A., Clark, D. A., Gershoff, E. T., Klump, K. L., & Hyde, L. W. (2021). Twin differences in harsh parenting predict youth's antisocial behavior. *Psychological Science, 32*(3), 395–409. https://doi.org/10.1177/0956797620968532
39. Gershoff, E. (2002). Corporal punishment by parents and associated child behaviors and experiences: A meta-analysis and theoretical review. *Psychological Bulletin, 128,* 530–579.

Others include Okuzono, S., Fujiwara, T., Kato, T., & Kawachi I. (2017). Spanking and subsequent behavioral problems in toddlers: A propensity score-matched, prospective study in Japan. *Child Abuse and Neglect, 69*, 62–71; Benjet, C., & Kazdin, A. E. (2003). Spanking children: The controversies, findings, and new directions. *Clinical Psychology Review, 23*, 197–224; Taylor, C. A., Manganello, J. A., Lee, S. J., & Rice, J. C. (2010). Mothers spanking of 3-year-old children and subsequent risk of children's aggressive behavior. *Pediatrics, 125*, 1057–1065; Altschul, I., Lee, S. J., & Gershoff, E. T. (2016). Hugs, not hits. Warmth and spanking as predictors of child social competence. *Journal of Marriage and the Family, 78*, 695–714. http://dx.doi.org/10.1111/jomf.12306; Durrant, J., & Ensom, R. (2012). Physical punishment of children: Lessons from 20 years of research. *CMAJ: Canadian Medical Association Journal, 184*, 1373–1377. http://dx.doi.org/10.1503/cmaj.101314; Gershoff, E. T., Lansford, J. E., Sexton, H. R., Davis-Kean, P., & Sameroff, A. J. (2012). Longitudinal links between spanking and children's externalizing behaviors in a national sample of White, Black Hispanic, and Asian American families. *Child Development, 83*, 838–843. http://dx.doi.org/10.1111/j.1467-8624.2011.01732.x; Gershoff, E. T., Font, S. A., Taylor, C. A., Foster, R. H., Garza, A. B., Olson-Dorff, D., Terreros, A., Nielsen-Parker, M., & Spector, L. (2016). Medical center staff attitudes about spanking, *Child Abuse & Neglect, 61*, 55–62, https://doi.org/10.1016/j.chiabu.2016.10.003; Gershoff, E. T., & Grogan-Kaylor, A. (2016). Corporal punishment by parents and its consequences for children: Old controversies and new meta-analyses. *Journal of Family Psychology, 30*, 453–469. http://dx.doi.org/10.1037/fam0000191

40. Thompson, R., Kaczor, K., Lorenz, D. J., Bennett, B. L., Meyers, G., & Pierce, M. C. (2017). Is the use of physical discipline associated with aggressive behaviors in young children? *Academic Pediatrics, 17*, 34–44; Ma, J., Grogan-Kaylor, A., & Lee, S. J. (2018). Associations of neighborhood disorganization and maternal spanking with children's aggression: A fixed-effects regression analysis. *Child Abuse & Neglect, 76*, 106–116; Gershoff, E. T., Sattler, K. M. P., & Ansari, A. (2018). Strengthening causal estimates for links between spanking and children's externalizing behavior problems. *Psychological Science, 29*(1) 110–120.

41. Cuartas, J. (2021). The effect of spanking on early social-emotional skills. *Child Development, 91*(4). https://doi.org/10.1111/cdev.13646

42. MacKenzie, M. J., Nicklas, E., Waldfogel, J., & Brooks-Gunn, J. (2012). Corporal punishment and child behavioural and cognitive outcomes through 5 years of age: Evidence from a contemporary urban birth cohort study. *Infant and Child Development, 21*, 3–33.

43. Lee, S. J., Altschul, I., & Gershoff, E. (2015). Wait until your father gets home: Mother's and fathers' spanking and development of child aggression. *Children and Youth Services Review, 52*, 158–166.

44. Lansford, J., Wager, L. B., Bates, J. E., Pettit, G. S., & Dodge, K. A. (2012). Forms of spanking and children's externalizing behaviors. *Family Relations, 61*(2), 224–236.

45. Straus, M. A., & Mouradian, V. E. (1998). Impulsive corporal punishment by mothers and antisocial behavior and impulsiveness of children. *Behavioral Sciences and the Law, 16*, 353–374.

46. MacKenzie, M. J., Nicklas, E., Brooks-Gunn, J., & Waldfogel, J. (2015). Spanking and children's externalizing behavior across the first decade of life: Evidence for transactional processes. *Journal of Youth Adolescence, 44*(3), 658–669.

47. Lansford, J. E., Wager, L. B., Bates, J. E., Pettit, G. S., & Dodge, K. A. (2012, April). Forms of spanking and children's externalizing behaviors. *Family Relations, 61*(2), 224–236.

48. Sheline, J. L., Skipper, B. J., & Broadhead, W. E. (1994). Risk factors for violent behavior in elementary school boys: Have you hugged your child today? *American Journal of Public Health, 84*(4), 661–663.
49. MacKenzie, M. J., Nicklas, E., Brooks-Gunn, J., & Waldfogel, J. (2014). Repeated exposure to high-frequency spanking and child externalizing behavior across the first decade: A moderating role for cumulative risk. *Child Abuse & Neglect, 38*, 1895–1901.
50. Boutwell, B. B., Franklin, C. A., Barnes, J. C., & Beaver, K. M. (2011). Physical punishment and childhood aggression: The role of gender and gene–environment interplay. *Aggressive Behavior, 37*, 559–568.
51. Gromoske, A. N., & Maguire-Jack, K. (2012). Transactional and cascading relations between early spanking and children's social-emotional development. *Sociological Abstracts, 74*(5), 1054–1068.
52. Gelles, R. J. (1974). *The Violent Home: A Study of Physical Aggression Between Husbands and Wives.* Beverly Hills, CA: Sage.
53. Carroll, J. C. (1977). The intergenerational transmission of family violence: Long-term effects of aggressive behavior. *Aggressive Behavior, 3*, 289–299.
54. Straus, M. A. (1990). Corporal punishment, child abuse, and wife-beating: What do they have in common? In M. A. Straus & R. J. Gelles (Eds.), *Physical Violence in American Families: Risk Factors and Adaptations to Violence in 8,145 Families* (pp. 403–424). New Brunswick, NJ: Transaction.
55. Kalmuss, D. S. (1984). The intergenerational transmission of marital aggression. *Journal of Marriage and the Family, 46*, 11–19.
56. Temple, J. R., Choi, H. J., Reuter, T., Wolfe, D., Taylor, C. A., Madigan, S., & Scott, L. E. (2018). Childhood corporal punishment and future perpetration of physical dating violence. *Journal of Pediatrics, 194*, 233–237.
57. Gage, A. J., & Silvestre, E. A. (2010). Maternal violence, victimization, and child physical punishment in Peru. *Child Abuse & Neglect, 34*, 523–533.
58. Straus, M., & Yodanis, C. L. (1996). Corporal punishment in adolescence and physical assaults in spouses in later life: What accounts for the link? *Journal of Marriage and Family, 58*(4), 825–841.
59. Tennant, F. S., Detels, R., & Clark, V. (1975). Some childhood antecedents of drug and alcohol abuse. *American Journal of Epidemiology, 102*(5), 377–387.
60. Hyland, M. E., & Alkhalaf, A. M. (2013). Beating and insulting children as a risk for adult cancer, cardiac disease and asthma. *Ben Whalley Journal of Behavioral Medicine, 36*, 632–640.
61. MacKenzie, M. J., Nicklas, E., Waldfogel, J., & Brooks-Gunn, J. (2012). Corporal punishment and child behavioural and cognitive outcomes through 5 years of age: Evidence from a contemporary urban birth cohort study. *Infant and Child Development, 21*, 3–33.
62. Font, S. A., & Cage, J. (2018). Dimensions of physical punishment and their associations with children's cognitive performance and school adjustment. *Child Abuse & Neglect, 75*, 29–40. http://dx.doi.org/10.1016/j.chiabu.2017.06.008
63. Turner, H. A., & Finkelhor, D. (1996). Corporal punishment as a stressor among youth. *Journal of Marriage and the Family, 58*(1), 155–166.
64. Turner, H. A., & Finkelhor, D. (1996). Corporal punishment as a stressor among youth. *Journal of Marriage and the Family, 58*(1), 155–166.
65. Afifi, T. O., Ford, D., Gershoff, E. T., Merrick, M., Grogan-Kaylor, A., Ports, K. A., MacMillan, H. L., Holden, G. W., Taylor, C. A., Lee, S. J., & Bennett, R. P. (2017). Spanking

and adult mental health impairment: The case for the designation of spanking as an adverse childhood experience. *Child Abuse & Neglect, 71*, 24–31. https://doi.org/10.1016/j.chiabu.2017.01.014

66. MacMillan, H. L., Boyle, M. H., Wong, M. Y.-Y., Duku, E. K., Fleming, J. E., & Walsh, C. A. (1999). Slapping and spanking in childhood and its association with lifetime prevalence of psychiatric disorders in a general population sample. *Canadian Medical Association Journal, 161*(7), 805–809.

67. Teicher, M. H., & Samson, J. A. (2016). Annual research review: Enduring neurobiological effects of childhood abuse and neglect. *Journal of Child Psychology and Psychiatry, 57*(3), 241–266.

68. Afifi, T. O., Mota, N. P., Dasiewicz, P., MacMillan, H. L., & Sareen, J. (2012). Physical punishment and mental disorders: Results from a nationally representative US sample. *Pediatrics, 130*(2), 184, 184–192.

69. Afifi, T. O., Mota, N. P., Dasiewicz, P., MacMillan, H. L., & Sareen, J. (2012). Physical punishment and mental disorders: Results from a nationally representative US sample. *Pediatrics, 130*(2), 184, 184–192.

70. Bandura, A. (1973). *Aggression: A Social Learning Analysis.* Englewood Cliffs, NJ: Prentice Hall.

71. Bandura, A. (1973). *Aggression: A Social Learning Analysis* (p. 148). Englewood Cliffs, NJ: Prentice Hall.

72. Bandura, A. (1973). *Aggression: A Social Learning Analysis* (p. 57). Englewood Cliffs, NJ: Prentice Hall.

73. Davitz, J. R. (1952). The effects of previous training on post-frustration behavior. *Journal of Abnormal and Social Psychology, 47*, 309–315.

74. Bandura, A. (1973). *Aggression: A Social Learning Analysis* (p. 53). Englewood Cliffs, NJ: Prentice Hall.

75. Nolen, J. L. (2020, May 26). *Bobo doll experiment. Encyclopedia Britannica.* https://www.britannica.com/event/Bobo-doll-experiment

76. Segment 50 Bandura's Bobo Doll Experiment; The Modeling of Aggression. Albert Bandura, Stanford University and Worth Publishers. https://www.youtube.com/watch?v=dmBqwWlJg8U

77. Van Der Kolk, B. (2014). *The Body Keeps the Score: Brain, Mind and Body in the Healing of Trauma* (p. 97). New York: Viking.

78. Grogan-Kaylor A., Ma, J., & Graham-Bermann, S. A. (2018). The case against physical punishment. *Current Opinion in Psychology, 19*, 22–27.

79. Van Der Kolk, B. (2014). *The Body Keeps the Score. Brain, Mind and Body in the Healing of Trauma* (p. 148). New York: Viking.

80. Larzelere, R. E. (2000). Child outcomes of nonabusive and customary physical punishment by parents: An updated literature review. *Clinical Child and Family Psychology Review, 3*(4).

81. Larzelere, R. E. (2000). Child outcomes of nonabusive and customary physical punishment by parents: An updated literature review. *Clinical Child and Family Psychology Review, 3*(4).

82. Powers, S. W., & Larzelere, R. E. Behavioral theory and corporal punishment. In M. Donnelly & M. A. Straus (Eds.), *Corporal Punishment of Children in Theoretical Perspective.* New Haven, CT: Yale University Press.

83. Baum, W .M., & Kupfer, A. S. (2005). Behavior analysis, evolutionary theory, and the corporal discipline of children. In M. Donnelly & M. A. Straus (Eds.), *Corporal Punishment of Children in Theoretical Perspective.* New Haven, CT: Yale University Press.

84. Powers, S. W., & Larzelere, R. E. (2005). Behavioral theory and corporal punishment. In M. Donnelly & M. A. Straus (Eds.), *Corporal Punishment of Children in Theoretical Perspective*. New Haven, CT: Yale University Press.

85. Larzelere, R. E., Sather, P. R., Schneider, W. N., Larson, D. B., & Pike, P. L. (1998). Punishment enhances reasoning's effectiveness as a disciplinary response to toddlers *Journal of Marriage and the Family, 60*(2), 388.

86. Larzelere, R. E. (2000). Child outcomes of nonabusive and customary physical punishment by parents: An updated literature review. *Clinical Child and Family Psychology Review, 3*(4).

87. Bourque, S., & Rohner, R. (1996). Children's perception of corporal punishment, care taker acceptance, and psychological adjustment. *Journal of Marriage and the Family, 58*(4), 842.

88. Gershoff, E. T. (2002). Corporal punishment by parents and associated child behaviors and experiences: A meta-analytic and theoretical review. *Psychological Bulletin, 128,* 539–579; Heilmann, A., Mehay, A., Watt, R. G., Kelly, Y., Durrant, J. E., van Turnhout, J., & Gershoff, E. T. (2021). Physical punishment and child outcomes: A narrative review of prospective studies. *Lancet, 398,* 355–364 https://doi.org/10.1016/S0140-6736(21)00582-1

89. Hart, B., & Risley, T. R. (1995). *Meaningful Differences in the Everyday Experiences of Young American Children* (p. 58). Baltimore: Paul H. Brookes.

90. Hart, B., & Risley, T. R. (1995). *Meaningful Differences in the Everyday Experiences of Young American Children* (p. 109). Baltimore: Paul H. Brookes.

91. Hemenway, D., Solnick, S., & Carter, J. (1994). Child rearing violence. *Child Abuse & Neglect, 18*(12), 1011–1020.

92. Kazdin, A. *The Kazdin Method of Parenting*. https://alankazdin.com/

93. Altschul, I., Lee, S. J., & Gershoff, E. T. (2016), Hugs, Not Hits: Warmth and Spanking as Predictors of Child Social Competence. *Family Relations, 78,* 695–714. https://doi.org/10.1111/jomf.12306

94. Gilligan, J. (2001). *Preventing Violence*. New York: Thames & Hudson.

95. Katz, J. (2012). *Violence Against Women: Its a Men's Issue*. Ted Talk. https://www.ted.com/talks/jackson_katz_violence_against_women_it_s_a_men_s_issue?language=en

96. Arain, M., Haque, M., Johal, L., Mathur, P., Nel, W., Rais, A., Sandhu, R., & Sharma, S. (2013). Maturation of the adolescent brain. *Neuropsychiatric disease and treatment, 9,* 449–461. https://doi.org/10.2147/NDT.S39776

97. Brown, B. (2012). *Daring Greatly: How the Courage to be Vulnerable Transforms the Way We Live, Love, Parent, and Lead*. New York: Penguin. p. 220.

98. Ansari, A., & Crosnoe, R. (2015). Children's elicitation of changes in parenting during the early childhood years. *Early Childhood Research Quarterly, 32,* 139–149.

99. Davis, P. W. (1999). Corporal punishment cessation: Social contexts and parents experiences. *Journal of Interpersonal Violence, 14*(5), 492–510.

100. Nagoski, E., & Nagoski, A. (2019). *Burnout: The Secret to Unlocking the Stress Cycle*. New York: Ballantine Books.

Chapter 5

1. Andero, A., & Stewart, A. (2002). Issue of corporal punishment: Re-examined. *Journal of Instructional Psychology, 29*(2), 90–96.

2. NBC Today. (2016, April 15). Paddling of 5-year-old by principal reignites debate over spanking.https://www.youtube.com/watch?v=djjpUcjWrLc

3. CNN. (2021, May 9). Florida State Attorney says no crime was committed when principal paddled 6 year old. https://www.cnn.com/2021/05/09/us/florida-school-student-padd led-state-attorney/index.html

4. Earle, A. M. (1993). *Child Life in Colonial Days*. Great Barrington, MA: Berkshire House.

5. Kratz, H. E. (1895). A bit of child study. *Journal of Education, 42*(8), 143.

6. *New York Times.* (1898). Spanking by electricity. https://www.nytimes.com/1898/02/14/ archives/spanking-by-electricity-kansas-has-invented-a-method-which-colorado.html

7. No Author. (1902). Corporal punishment in twenty-five American cities. *Journal of Education, 56*(21), 346.

8. No Author. (1902). Corporal punishment in twenty-five American cities. *Journal of Education, 56*(21), 346.

9. Harris, T. H., Glenn, C. B., Cooley, R. L., & Stetson, P. C. (1929, October 21). Is corporal punishment still necessary? *Journal of Education, 110*(13), 321–322.

10. Block, N. A. (2013). *Breaking the Paddle: Ending School Corporal Punishment.* Published by Nadine A. Block.

11. Welsh, R. S., et al. (1976). The Supreme Court spanking ruling: an issue in debate (p. 2). Paper presented at the Annual Convention of the American Psychological Association, Chicago, April 13 and 14, 1976.

12. Anderson, K. A., & Anderson, D. E. (1976). Psychologists and spanking. *Journal of Clinical Child Psychology, 5*(2), 46–49.

13. Anderson, K. A., & Anderson, D. E. (1976). Psychologists and spanking. *Journal of Clinical Child Psychology, 5*(2), 46–49, quote from p. 49.

14. Welsh, R. S., et al. (1976). The Supreme Court spanking ruling: An issue in debate (p. 8). Paper presented at the Annual Convention of the American Psychological Association, Chicago, April 13 and 14, 1976.

15. Welsh, R. S., et al. (1976). The Supreme Court spanking ruling: an issue in debate (p. 22). Paper presented at the Annual Convention of the American Psychological Association, Chicago, April 13 and 14, 1976.

16. Welsh, R. S., et al. (1976). The Supreme Court spanking ruling: an issue in debate (p. 22). Paper presented at the Annual Convention of the American Psychological Association, Chicago, April 13 and 14, 1976.

17. Welsh, R. S., et al. (1976). The Supreme Court spanking ruling: an issue in debate (p. 2). Paper presented at the Annual Convention of the American Psychological Association, Chicago, April 13 and 14, 1976.

18. Welsh, R. S., et al. (1976). The Supreme Court spanking ruling: an issue in debate (p. 17). Paper presented at the Annual Convention of the American Psychological Association, Chicago, April 13 and 14, 1976.

19. Welsh, R. S., et al. (1976). The Supreme Court spanking ruling: an issue in debate (p. 68). Paper presented at the Annual Convention of the American Psychological Association, Chicago, April 13 and 14, 1976.

20. Hyman, I. (1990). *Reading, Writing and the Hickory Stick: The Appalling Story of Physical and Psychological Abuse in American Schools.* Lexington, MA: Lexington Books.

21. Welsh, R. S., et al. (1976). The Supreme Court spanking ruling: an issue in debate (p. 5). Paper presented at the Annual Convention of the American Psychological Association, Chicago, April 13 and 14, 1976.

22. The *Ingraham v. Wright* case is a compilation of several sources: Greven, P. J. (1990). *Spare the Child: The Religious Roots of Punishment and the Psychological Impact of Physical Abuse* (pp. 100–101). New York: Vintage Books; Hyman, I. (1990). *Reading, Writing and the Hickory Stick: The Appalling Story of Physical and Psychological Abuse in American Schools.* Lexington, MA: Lexington Books; Gershoff, E., & Font, S. (2016). Corporal punishment in U.S. public schools: Prevalence, disparities in use, and status in state and federal policy. *Social Policy Report, 30*(1). www.srcd.org/publications/social-policy-report

23. Greven, P. J. (1990). *Spare the Child: The Religious Roots of Punishment and the Psychological Impact of Physical Abuse* (pp. 100–101). New York: Vintage Books.

24. Sidman, M. (2001). *Coercion and It's Fallout.* Boston: Authors Cooperative.

25. Courthouse News Service. (2011, August 25). Boy says school paddling broke his jaw. https://www.courthousenews.com/boy-says-school-paddling-broke-his-jaw/

26. www.nadineblock.com

27. Block, N. A. (2013). *Breaking the Paddle: Ending School Corporal Punishment.* Published by Nadine A. Block.

28. Block, N. A. (2013). *Breaking the Paddle: Ending School Corporal Punishment.* Published by Nadine A. Block

29. PTA.org Resolution. Adopted by 1985 Convention Delegates.

30. PTA.org Resolution: Corporal Punishment.

31. Hyman, I. (1990). *Reading, Writing and the Hickory Stick: The Appalling Story of Physical and Psychological Abuse in American Schools.* Lexington, MA: Lexington Books.

32. Center for Effective Discipline. (2014). Paddling versus ACT scores—A retrospective analysis. http://www.stophitting.com/index.php?page=paddlingvsact

33. Gershoff, E. T., Purtell, K. M., & Holas, I. (2015). *Corporal Punishment in US Public Schools: Legal Precedents, Current Practices and Legal Policy.* New York: Springer.

34. Peterson, E. (2005, March 6). Discipline policy leads to quandary. Mother says school should not make her spank 6-year-old son. *Chicago Daily Herald.*

35. Sales of "Make Kids Great Again" spanking paddles draw criticism, praise. https://kutv.com/news/offbeat/sales-of-make-kids-great-again-spanking-paddles-draw-criticism-praise

36. US Government Accountability Office, Report to Congressional Requesters. (2018). K-12 education discipline disparities for black students, boys, and students with disabilities. https://www.gao.gov/assets/700/690828.pdf and Richardson, R. C., & Evans, E. T. (1992). African-American Males: Endangered Species and the Most Paddled. Annual Meeting of the Louisiana Association of Multicultural Education.

37. Abrams, J. The Board of Education: A documentary about corporal punishment in US public schools. Wide Open Camera. https://stopspanking.org/resources/end-school-paddling/.

38. Gershoff, E. T., Purtell, K. M., & Holas, I. (2015). *Corporal Punishment in U.S. Public Schools: Legal Precedents, Current Practices, and Future Policy.* New York: Springer; Hyman, I. (1990). *Reading, Writing and the Hickory Stick: The Appalling Story of Physical and Psychological Abuse in American Schools.* Lexington, MA: Lexington Books.

39. Hyman, I. (1990). *Reading, Writing and the Hickory Stick: The Appalling Story of Physical and Psychological Abuse in American Schools.* Lexington, MA: Lexington Books.

40. Gershoff, E. T., Purtell, K. M., & Holas, I. (2015). *Corporal Punishment in U.S. Public Schools: Legal Precedents, Current Practices, and Future Policy.* New York: Springer.

41. Civil Rights Data Collection. 2013–2014 data notes. (No page number for quote) https://ocrdata.ed.gov/assets/downloads/2013-2014/Data-Notes-CRDC-2013-14.pdf

42. Gershoff, E. T., Purtell, K. M., & Holas, I. (2015). *Corporal Punishment in U.S. Public Schools: Legal Precedents, Current Practices, and Future Policy.* New York: Springer.

43. Gershoff, E., & Font, S. (2016). Corporal punishment in U.S. public schools: Prevalence, disparities in use, and status in state and federal policy. *Social Policy Report, 30*(1). www.srcd.org/publications/social-policy-report

44. US Government Accountability Office, Report to Congressional Requesters. (2018). K-12 education discipline disparities for black students, boys, and students with disabilities. https://www.gao.gov/assets/700/690828.pdf

45. Devries, K. M., Child, J. C., Allen, E., Walakira, E., Parkes, J., & Naker, D. (2014). School violence, mental health, and educational performance in Uganda. *Pediatrics, 133*(1), e129–e137. https://doi.org/10.1542/peds.2013-2007; Baker-Henningham, H., Meeks-Gardner, J., Chang, S., & Walker, S. (2009). Experiences of violence and deficits in academic achievement among urban primary school children in Jamaica. *Child Abuse & Neglect, 33*(5), 296–306. https://doi.org/10.1016/ j.chiabu.2008.05.01; Talwar, V., Carlson, S. M., & Lee, K. (2011). Effects of a punitive environment on children's executive functioning: A natural experiment. *Social Development, 20*(4), 805–824. https://doi.org/10.1111/j.1467-9507.2011.00617.x

46. Youssef, R. M., Attia, M. S., & Kamel, M. I. (1999). Violence among schoolchildren in Alexandria. *Eastern Mediterranean Health Journal, 5*(2), 282–298; Ani, C. C., & Grantham-McGregor, S. (1998). Family and personal characteristics of aggressive Nigerian boys: Differences from and similarities with western findings. *Journal of Adolescent Health, 23*(5), 311–317. https://doi.org/10.1016/s1054-139x(98)00031-7

47. DeNisco, A. (2013, June). Paddling makes a comeback in Florida schools. District Administration (p. 16). Educators Reference Complete. http://link.galegroup.com/apps/doc/A334844139/PROF?u=clic_augsburg&sid=PROF&xid=cca379ab

48. Block, N. A. (2013). *Breaking the Paddle: Ending School Corporal Punishment.* Published by Nadine A. Block.

49. Martin, M., (2008). To spank or not to spank? Moms discuss discipline. Opposing viewpoints in context. Tell Me More. National Public Radio.

50. Southern Poverty Law Center and the Center of Civil Rights Remedies. (2019). *The striking outlier: The persistent, painful and problematic practice of corporal punishment in schools.*

51. Gershoff, E. T., Purtell, K. M., & Holas, I. (2015) *Corporal Punishment in U.S. Public Schools: Legal Precedents, Current Practices, and Future Policy.* New York: Springer.

52. Southern Poverty Law Center and the Center of Civil Rights Remedies. (2019). The striking outlier: The persistent, painful and problematic practice of corporal punishment in schools.

53. Gershoff, E. T., Purtell, K. M., & Holas, I. (2015) *Corporal Punishment in U.S. Public Schools: Legal Precedents, Current Practices, and Future Policy.* New York: Springer.

54. Kennedy, B. L., Murphy, A. S., & Jordan, A. (2017). Title I middle school administrators' beliefs and choices about using corporal punishment and exclusionary discipline (p. 258). *American Journal of Education, 123*, 243–280.

55. Han, S. (2014). Corporal punishment and student outcomes in rural schools. *Educational Research for Policy and Practice, 13*(3), 221–231. https://doi.org/10.1007/s10671-014-9161-0

56. Czumbil, M. R., & Hyman, I. A. (1997). What happens when corporal punishment is legal? *Journal of Interpersonal Violence, 12*, 309–315.

57. Gershoff, E., & Font, S. (2016). Corporal punishment in U.S. public schools: Prevalence, disparities in use, and status in state and federal policy. *Social Policy Report, 30*(1). www.srcd.org/publications/social-policy-report

58. Van Der Kolk, B. (2014). *The Body Keeps the Score. Brain, Mind and Body in the Healing of Trauma* (p. 353). New York: Viking.

59. Amiker, F. (2015, March 9). Video shows girl held down, paddled in school. https://www.news4jax.com/news/2015/03/10/video-shows-girl-held-down-paddled-in-school/

60. Patton, S. (2017). *Spare the Kids: Why Whupping Children Won't Save Black America* (p. 116). Boston: Beacon Press.

61. Crain, T. P. (2016, September 12). Why did Alabama paddle 19,000 students in one school year? *Birmingham Real Time News*. https://www.al.com/news/birmingham/2016/09/alabama_schools_paddling.html

62. de Brey, C., Musu, L., McFarland, J., Wilkinson-Flicker, S., Diliberti, M., Zhang, A., Branstetter, C., & Wang, X. (2019). Status and trends in the education of racial and ethnic groups 2018 (NCES 2019-038). Washington, DC: US Department of Education, National Center for Education Statistics. https://nces.ed.gov/pubsearch/

63. Menakem, R. (2017). *My grandmother's hands: Racialized trauma and the pathways to mending our hearts and bodies.* Las Vegas, NV: Central Recovery Press.

64. Riddle, T., & Sinclair, S. (2019). Racial disparities in school-based disciplinary actions are associated with county-level rates of racial bias. *Proceedings of the National Academy of Sciences, 116*(17), 8255–8260.

65. Block, N. A. (2013). *Breaking the Paddle: Ending School Corporal Punishment.* Published by Nadine A. Block..

66. US Government Accountability Office, Report to Congressional Requesters. (2018). K-12 education discipline disparities for black students, boys, and students with disabilities. https://www.gao.gov/assets/700/690828.pdf

67. Green, E. (2018, March). Why are Black students punished so often? Minnesota confronts a national quandary. *New York Times*. https://www.nytimes.com/2018/03/18/us/politics/school-discipline-disparities-white-Black-students.html

68. Balingit, M. (2018, April 24). Racial disparities in children are growing, federal data show. *Washington Post*. https://www.washingtonpost.com/local/education/racial-disparities-in-school-discipline-are-growing-federal-data-shows/2018/04/24/67b5d2b8-47e4-11e8-827e-190efaf1f1ee_story.html

69. Gershoff, E. T., Sattler, K. M., & Holden, G. W. (2019). School corporal punishment and its associations with achievement and adjustment. *Journal of Applied Developmental Psychology, 63*, 1–8.

70. Gershoff, E., & Font, S. (2016). Corporal punishment in U.S. public schools: Prevalence, disparities in use, and status in state and federal policy. *Social Policy Report, 30*(1). www.srcd.org/publications/social-policy-report

71. Melisizwe, T. (2020, July 10). Dignity in Schools campaign statement on anti-Black violence and education justice. https://dignityinschools.org/dignity-in-schools-campaign-statement-on-anti-Black-violence-and-education-justice/

72. Melisizwe, T. (2020, July 10). Dignity in Schools campaign statement on anti-Black violence and education justice. https://dignityinschools.org/dignity-in-schools-campaign-statement-on-anti-Black-violence-and-education-justice/

73. US Department of Education. https://www.ed.gov/news/press-releases/king-sends-letter-states-calling-end-corporal-punishment-schools

74. Martin, M. (2008). To spank or not to spank? Moms discuss discipline. Opposing viewpoints in context. Tell Me More. National Public Radio.
75. Conte, A. E. (2000). In loco parentis: Alive and well. *Education, 121*, 195–200.
76. Heekes, S. L., Kruger, C. B., & Lester, S. N., & Ward., C. L. (2022) A systematic review of corporal punishment in schools: global prevalence and correlates. *Trauma, Violence and Abuse, 23*(1), 52–72. https://doi.org/10.1177/1524838020925787
77. Global Initiative to End All Corporal Punishment of Children. (2018). Global Report. www.Endcorporalpunishment.org
78. Florida still spanking its schoolkids: Who's getting hit the most. https://www.palmbeachp ost.com/news/news/state-regional-education/florida-still-spanking-its-schoolkids-whos-getting/nkFt6/?&_ga=2.159664893.1984107014.1596333010-1027225632.1594296990
79. All Information for H.R.727—Ending Corporal Punishment in Schools Act of 2019. https://www.congress.gov/bill/116th-congress/house-bill/727/all-info
80. H.R. 1234—117th Congress: Ending Corporal Punishment in Schools Act of 2021. www. GovTrack.us; https://www.govtrack.us/congress/bills/117/hr1234.
81. Global Initiative to End All Corporal Punishment. (2018). Global Report 2018: Progress Towards Ending Corporal Punishment of Children.
82. https://endcorporalpunishment.org/sri-lanka-supreme-court-judgment-condemns-corporal-punishment-in-schools/
83. End Violence Against Children, Safe to Learn. https://www.end-violence.org/safe-to-learn
84. Gershoff, E., & Font, S. (2016). Corporal punishment in U.S. public schools: Prevalence, disparities in use, and status in state and federal policy. *Social Policy Report, 30*(1). www. srcd.org/publications/social-policy-report
85. Welsh, R. S., et al. (1976). The Supreme Court spanking ruling: An issue in debate (p. 71). Paper presented at the Annual Convention of the American Psychological Association, Chicago, April 13 and 14, 1976.

Chapter 6

1. Andero, A., & Stewart, A. (2002). Issue of corporal punishment: Re-examined. *Journal of Instructional Psychology, 29*(2), 90–96.
2. Gerhardt, S. (2004). *Why Love Matters: How Affection Shapes a Baby's Brain.* New York: Brunner-Routledge.
3. Fairbanks, L. A., & McGuire, M. T. (2005). Parent-offspring conflict and corporal punishment in primates. In M. Donnelly & M. A. Straus (Eds.), *Corporal Punishment of Children in Theoretical Perspective* (pp. 21–40). New Haven: Yale University Press.
4. Fairbanks, L. A., & McGuire, M. T. (2005). Parent-offspring conflict and corporal punishment in primates. In M. Donnelly & M. A. Straus (Eds.), *Corporal Punishment of Children in Theoretical Perspective* (pp. 21–40). New Haven: Yale University Press.
5. Crittenden, P. M. (2005). The origins of physical punishment: An ethological/attachment perspective on the use of physical punishment by human parents. In M. Donnelly & M. A. Straus (Eds.), *Corporal Punishment of Children in Theoretical Perspective* (pp. 73–90). New Haven: Yale University Press.
6. Fairbanks, L. A., & McGuire, M. T. (2005). Parent-offspring conflict and corporal punishment in primates. In M. Donnelly & M. A. Straus (Eds.), *Corporal Punishment of Children in Theoretical Perspective* (pp. 21–40). New Haven: Yale University Press.

7. Pinker, S. (2011). The Better Angels of Our Nature: Why Violence Has Declined (p. 431). New York: Penguin.

8. Fairbanks, L. A., & McGuire, M. T. (2005). Parent-offspring conflict and corporal punishment in primates. In M. Donnelly & M. A. Straus (Eds.), *Corporal Punishment of Children in Theoretical Perspective* (pp. 21–40). New Haven: Yale University Press.

9. Fairbanks, L. A., & McGuire, M. T. (2005). Parent-offspring conflict and corporal punishment in primates. In M. Donnelly & M. A. Straus (Eds.), *Corporal Punishment of Children in Theoretical Perspective* (pp. 21–40). New Haven: Yale University Press.

10. Pinker, S. (2011). *The Better Angels of Our Nature: Why Violence Has Declined* (p. 394). New York: Penguin.

11. Pinker, S. (2011). *The Better Angels of Our Nature: Why Violence Has Declined* (p. 394). New York: Penguin.

12. Crittenden, P. M. (2005). The origins of physical punishment: An ethological/attachment perspective on the use of physical punishment by human parents. In M. Donnelly & M. A. Straus (Eds.), *Corporal Punishment of Children in Theoretical Perspective* (pp. 73–90). New Haven: Yale University Press.

13. Ribeiro, C. S., Coelho, L., & Magalhaes, T. (2016). Comparing corporal punishment and children's exposure to violence between caregivers: Towards better diagnosis and prevention of intrafamilial physical abuse of children. *Journal of Forensic and Legal Medicine, 38*, 11–17.

14. Runyan, D. K., Shankar, V., Hassan, F., Hunter, W. M., Jain, D., Paula, C. S., Bangdiwala, S. I., Ramiro, L. S., Munoz, S. R., Vizcarra, B., & Bordin, I. A. (2010). International variations in harsh child discipline. *Pediatrics, 126*(3), e701–711.

15. United Nations Children's Fund. (2014). *Hidden in Plain Sight*. New York: UNICEF; Know Violence in Childhood. (2017). *Ending Violence in Childhood*. Global Report 2017. New Delhi: Know Violence in Childhood.

16. Lansford, J. E., Alampay, L. P., Al-Hassan, S., Bacchini, D., Bombi, A. S., Bornstein, M. H., Chang, L., Deater-Deckard, K., Di Giunta, L., Dodge, K. A., Oburu, P., Pastorelli, C., Runyan, D., Skinner, A. T., Sorbring, E., Tapanya, S., Uribe Tirado, L. M., & Zelli, A. (2010). Corporal punishment of children in nine countries as a function of child gender and parent gender. *International Journal of Pediatrics, 2010*, 1–12. doi:10.1155/2010/672780.

17. Vittrup, B., & Holden, G. W. (2010). Children's assessments of corporal punishment and other disciplinary practices: The role of age, race, SES, and exposure to spanking. *Journal of Applied Developmental Psychology, 31*, 211–220.

18. Lansford, J. E., et al. (2010). Corporal punishment of children in nine countries as a function of child gender and parent gender. *International Journal of Pediatrics, 2010*, 672780.

19. Cappa, C., & Khan, S. M. (2011). Understanding caregivers attitudes towards corporal punishment of children: Evidence from 34 low-and middle-income countries. *Child Abuse & Neglect, 35*, 1009–1021.

20. Convention on the Rights of the Child, United Nations Human Rights, Office of the High Commissioner. https://www.ohchr.org/en/professionalinterest/pages/crc.aspx

21. Janson, S. (2018). Tracking progress towards non-violent childhoods: Measuring changes in attitudes and behavior to achieve an end to corporal punishment. Council of the Baltic Sea States Secretariat Slussplan 9, Stockholm, Sweden.

22. Missildine, W. H. (1963). *Your Inner Child of the Past*. New York: Simon & Schuster.

23. Pace, G. T., Lee, S. J., & Grogan-Kaylor, A. (2019). Spanking and young children's socioemotional development in low- and middle-income countries. *Child Abuse & Neglect,*

88, 84–95; Cuartas, J. (2021). Corporal punishment and early childhood development in 49 low- and middle-income countries. *Child Abuse & Neglect, 120*, 105205.

24. Levinson, D. (1989). *Family Violence in Cross Cultural Perspective*. Newbury Park: Sage.

25. Lansford, J. E., Alampay, L. P., Al-Hassan, S., Bacchini, D., Bombi, A. S., Bornstein, M. H., Chang, L., Deater-Deckard, K., Di Giunta, L., Dodge, K. A., Oburu, P., Pastorelli, C., Runyan, D., Skinner, A. T., Sorbring, E., Tapanya, S., Uribe Tirado, L. M., & Zelli, A. (2010). Corporal punishment of children in nine countries as a function of child gender and parent gender. *International Journal of Pediatrics, 2010*, 1–12 doi:10.1155/2010/672780.

26. Ember, C., & Ember M. (2005). Explaining corporal punishment of children: A cross cultural study. *American Anthropologist, 107*(4), 609–619.

27. Chang, I. J., Pettit, R. W., & Katsurada, E. (2006). Where and when to spank: A comparison between US and Japanese college students. *Journal of Family Violence, 21*, 281–286.

28. Wainryb, C. (1993). The application of moral judgements to other cultures: Relativism and universality. *Child Development, 64*(3), 924–933.

29. Lansford, J. E., Dodge, K. A., Malone, P. S., Bacchini, D., Zelli, A., et al. (2005). Physical discipline and child adjustment: Cultural normativeness as a moderator. *Child Development, 76*(6), 1234–1246.

30. Heilmann, A., Mehay, A., Watt, R. G., Kelly, Y., Durrant, J. E., van Turnhout, J., & Gershoff, E. T. (2021). Physical punishment and child outcomes: A narrative review of prospective studies. *Lancet, 398*, 355–364. https://doi.org/10.1016/S0140-6736(21)00582-1

31. *Prince George Citizen*. (2000, July 14). How'd you like a spank, dad? Youth debaters urge repeal of law which permits hitting kids. Canadian Press.

32. Government of Canada, Department of Justice, Criminal Law and Managing Children's Behaviour. https://www.justice.gc.ca/eng/rp-pr/cj-jp/fv-vf/mcb-cce/index.html

33. *Prince George Citizen*. (2000, July 14). How'd you like a spank, dad? Youth debaters urge repeal of law which permits hitting kids. Canadian Press.

34. Durrant, J. E., Fallon, B., Lefebvre, R., & Allan, K. (2017). Defining reasonable force: Does it advance child protection? *Child Abuse & Neglect, 71*, 32–43.

35. YouTube. (2016). Hollywood encouraged the spanking and abuse of women onscreen. https://www.youtube.com/watch?v=K1sr-NjFUEE

36. Pimm, G. (n.d.). *The Corporal Punishment of Women: A True Historical and Contemporary Record*. Self-published.

37. Schmidt, S. (2018, January 3). Alabama newspaper executive admits spanking a female employee. *Washington Post*. https://www.chicagotribune.com/nation-world/ct-anniston-star-sexual-assault-20180103-story.html

38. CNN. (2019, December). Runner who slapped a reporter's backside on live TV says he's sorry. https://www.cnn.com/2019/12/13/us/runner-hits-reporter-backside-apology-trnd/index.html

39. Straus, M. A., Gelles, R. J., & Steinmetz, S. K. (1980). *Behind Closed Doors: Violence in the American Family*. New York: Anchor Books.

40. Patton, S. (2017). *Spare the Kids: Why Whupping Children Won't Save Black America*. Boston: Beacon Press.

41. The Global Initiative to End All Corporal Punishment of Children. (2020, January 4). Family Violence Briefing. Committee on the Elimination of Discrimination Against Women.

42. Becker, J. (2021). The evolution of the children's rights movement. In J. Todres & S. M. King (Eds.), *The Oxford Handbook of Children's Rights Law* (pp. 35–36). New York: Oxford University Press.

43. Korbin, J. E., & Krugman, R. D. (2015). *Child Maltreatment: Contemporary Issues in Research and Policy* (p. 545). New York: Springer.

44. Pais, M. S. (2021). Placing children's freedom from violence at the heart of the policy agenda. In J. Todres & S. M. King (Eds.), *The Oxford Handbook of Children's Rights Law* (p. 307). New York: Oxford University Press.

45. UN Committee on the Rights of the Child, General Comment No. 8 (2006) on "The right of the child to protection from corporal punishment and other cruel or degrading forms of punishment" (arts. 19; 28, para. 2; and 37, inter alia), paras. 27–28.

46. Durrant, J. E. (2008). Physical punishment, culture, and rights: Current issues for professionals. *Journal of Developmental Behavioral Pediatrics, 29*(1), 55–66.

47. Wainryb, C. (1993). The application of moral judgements to other cultures: Relativism and universality. *Child Development, 64*(3), 924–933.

48. Rowland, A., Gerry F., & Stanton, M. Physical punishment of children: Time to end the defence of reasonable chastisement in the UK, USA and Australia (2017). *International Journal of Children's Rights, 25*, 165–195.

49. The Global Initiative to End All Corporal Punishment of Children. (2018). Ending legalised violence against children by 2030: Progress towards prohibition and elimination of corporal punishment in pathfinder countries.

50. Prohibiting violent punishment of girls and boys—A key element in ending family violence. http://endcorporalpunishment.org/wp-content/uploads/thematic/Family-violence-briefing-2015.pdf. The Global Initiative To End All Corporal Punishment of Children.

51. Henry, A., & Lenihan, T., & Global Initiative to End All Corporal Punishment of Children. (2018). Ensuring non-violent childhoods: Guidance on Implementing the prohibition of corporal punishment in domestic settings. Council of the Baltic Sea States Secretariat: Stockholm, Sweden.

52. Gilligan, J. (2001). *Preventing Violence.* New York: Thames & Hudson.

53. Davis, P. W. (2003). *Social Problems Constructionist Readings.* Hawthorne, New York: Aldine de Gruyter.

54. Haldorsson, O. L. (2018). Building supportive societies for nonviolent childhoods: Awareness raising campaigns to achieve an end to corporal punishment. Council of the Baltic Sea States Secretariat Slussplan 9, Stockholm, Sweden.

55. Janson, S. (2018). Tracking progress towards non-violent childhoods: Measuring changes in attitudes and behaviors to achieve and end to corporal punishment. Council of the Baltic Sea States Secretariat Slussplan 9, Stockholm, Sweden.

56. Henry, A., & Lenihan, T. (2018). A step by step guide to implementing the Convention on the Rights of the Child. Global Initiative to End All Corporal Punishment of Children. Council of the Baltic Seas, Stockholm, Sweden.

57. Lansford, J. E., Cappa, C., Putnick, D. L., Bornstein, M. H., Deater-Deckard, K., & Bradley, R. H. (2017). Change over time in parents beliefs about and reports use of corporal punishment in eight countries with and without legal bans. *Child Abuse & Neglect, 71*, 44–55.

58. Educating Matters (2021). National spank out day—Why smacking doesn't work and what to do instead. https://www.educatingmatters.co.uk/blog/national-spank-out-day-why-smacking-does-not-work-what-to-do-instead/; Stop Abuse Campaign. (2021) April 30th is No Spank Day. https://stopabusecampaign.org/2018/04/06/april-30th-is-no-spank-day/

59. Rowland, A., Gerry F., & Stanton, M. (2017). Physical punishment of children time to end the defence of reasonable chastisement in the UK, USA and Australia. *International Journal of Children's Rights, 25*, 165–195.

60. United Nations. (2020, January 3). Sustainable development goals, knowledge platform. Violence against children. https://sustainabledevelopment.un.org/topics/violenceagainstc hildren

61. Mahatma Gandhi. In Ratcliffe, S. (Ed.), *Oxford Essential Quotations*. New York: Oxford University Press. https://www.oxfordreference.com/view/10.1093/acref/9780191866 692.001.0001/q-oro-ed6-00004716.

62. Global Initiative to End All Corporal Punishment of Children. (2015). Ending violent punishment of children: A foundation of a world free from fear and violence. http://endcorpora lpunishment.org/wp-content/uploads/thematic/SDG-indicators-on-violent-punishment-briefing.pdf

63. Elgar, F. J., Donnelly, P. D., Michaelson, V., et al. (2018). Corporal punishment bans and physical fighting in adolescents: an ecological study of 88 countries. *BMJ Open, 8*, e021616.

64. The Global Initiative to End All Corporal Punishment of Children. (2018). Ending legalised violence against children by 2030: Progress towards prohibition and elimination of corporal punishment in pathfinder countries.

65. Collins, R. (2005). Conflict Theory of Corporal Punishment. In M. Donnelly & M. A. Straus (Eds.), *Corporal Punishment of Children in Theoretical Perspective*. New Haven: Yale University Press.

66. Wilkins, W., Myers, L., Kuehl, T., Bauman, A., & Hertz, M. (2018). Connecting the dots: State Health department approaches to addressing shared risk and protective factors across multiple forms of violence. *Journal of Public Health Management and Practices, 24*(Suppl. 1), S32–S41.

67. Gracia, E., & Herrero, J. (2008). Beliefs in the necessity of corporal punishment of children and public perceptions of child physical abuse as a social problem. *Child Abuse & Neglect, 32*, 1058–1062.

68. Hazel, N., Ghate, D., Creighton, S., Field, J., & Finch, S. (2003). Violence against children: Threshold of acceptance for physical punishment in a normative study of parents, children and discipline (pp. 49–68). In E. Stanko (Ed.), *The Meanings of Violence*. London: Routledge.

69. Hazel, N., Ghate, D. Creighton, S., Field, J., & Finch, S. (2003). Violence against children: Threshold of acceptance for physical punishment in a normative study of parents, children and discipline. In E. Stanko (Ed.), *The Meanings of Violence* (pp. 49–68; quote from 63). London: Routledge.

70. Hite, S. (1994). *The Hite Report on the Family: Growing up Under Patriarchy* (p. 360). New York: Grove Press.

71. Hite, S. (1994). *The Hite Report on the Family: Growing up Under Patriarchy*. New York: Grove Press.

72. Miller, A. (1983). *For Your Own Good: Hidden Cruelty in Child Rearing and the Roots of Violence*. New York: Farrar, Straus, Giroux.

73. Patton, S. (2017). *Spare the Kids: Why Whupping Children Won't Save Black America*. Boston: Beacon Press.

74. Greven, P. J. (1990). *Spare the Child: The Religious Roots of Punishment and the Psychological Impact of Physical Abuse* (p. 122). New York: Vintage Books.

75. Freeman, M. (2021). Taking children's human rights seriously. In J. Todres & S. M. King (Eds.), *The Oxford Handbook of Children's Rights Laws* (p. 52). New York: Oxford University Press.

Chapter 7

1. Appleton, R. (2018). Arambula charged with child abuse, takes leave from California Assembly. *The Fresno Bee*. https://www.fresnobee.com/news/local/crime/article227469 979.html

2. Appleton, R. (2018, December 13). Fresno police chief adds details on Arambula arrest in the wake of assemblyman's explanation. https://www.sacbee.com/news/california/artic le223079675.html

3. GV Wire (2019, March 12). Assemblyman Arambula Goes on Leave After Child Cruelty Charges Filed. https://gvwire.com/2019/03/12/da-charges-assemblyman-arambula-with-child-cruelty/

4. Associated Press, (December, 2018). Lawmaker arrested for child cruelty says he spanked daughter.

5. *Fresno Bee*. (2019, May 16). Arambula found not guilty in child abuse case. He returns to capitol Monday. https://www.fresnobee.com/news/local/article230475269.html

6. Education in Action. (1927). Parents given spanking hints. *Journal of Education, 106*(16), 420–422.

7. Dodson, F. (1970). *How to Parent* (p. 209). New Jersey: Castle Books.

8. Dodson, F. (1970). *How to Parent* (pp. 208–209). New Jersey: Castle Books.

9. Gochros, J. S. (1977). *Only Spank When You're Angry. American Baby Magazine, 39*, 34–35.

10. Radl, S. L., (1980). American baby: To spank or not to spank. American *Association for Maternal and Child Health, 42*, 42.

11. Martin, M. (2008). To spank or not to spank? Moms discuss discipline. Opposing Viewpoints in Context. Tell Me More. National Public Radio.

12. Furman, E. (1993). *Toddlers and Mothers*. Madison, CT: International Universities Press.

13. https://christianblogs.christianet.com/1236214910.htm

14. Gerhardt, S. (2004). *Why Love Matters: How Affection Shapes a Baby's Brain*. New York: Brunner-Routledge.

15. Dunn, J., & Plomin, R. (1991). *Separate Lives: Why Siblings are So Different*. New York: Basic Books.

16. Missildine, W. H. (1963). *Your Inner Child of the Past* (pp. 26–29). New York: Simon & Schuster.

17. MacKenzie, M. J., Nicklas, E., Waldfogel, J., & Brooks-Gunn, J. (2012). Corporal punishment and child behavioural and cognitive outcomes through 5 years of age: Evidence from a contemporary urban birth cohort study. *Infant and Child Development, 21*, 3–33.

18. Gladwell, M. (2005). *Blink: The Power of Thinking Without Thinking*. New York: Little, Brown.

19. Ross, L. (1977). The intuitive psychologist and his shortcomings: Distortions in the attribution process. *Advances in Experimental Social Psychology, 10*, 173–220.

20. Day, R. D., Peterson, G. W., McCracken, C. (1998). Predicting spanking of younger and older children by mothers and fathers, *Journal of Marriage and the Family, 60*, 79–94.

21. Crouch, J. L., Irwin, L. M., Milner, J. S., Skowronski, J. J., Rutledge, E., & Davila, A. L. (2017). Do hostile attributions and negative affect explain the association between authoritarian beliefs and harsh parenting? *Child Abuse & Neglect, 67*, 13–21.

22. Sidman, M. (2001). *Coercion and It's Fallout*. Boston: Authors Cooperative.

23. Dowrick, S. (2005) *Choosing Happiness: Life and Soul Essentials*. New York: Penguin.

24. Patton, S. (2017). *Spare the Kids: Why Whupping Children Won't Save Black America* (p. 148). Boston: Beacon Press.

25. Samalin, N. (1991). *Love and Anger: The Parental Dilemma* (p. 58). New York: Penguin Books.

26. Nagoski, E., & Nagoski, A. (2019). *Burnout: The Secret to Unlocking the Stress Cycle*. New York: Ballantine Books.

27. Nagoski, E., & Nagoski, A. (2019). *Burnout: The Secret to Unlocking the Stress Cycle*. New York: Ballantine Books.

28. Mikolajczak, M., Brianda, M. E., Avalosse, H., & Roskam, I. (2018). Consequences of parental burnout: Its specific effect on child neglect and violence, *Child Abuse & Neglect, 80,* 134–145. https://doi.org/10.1016/j.chiabu.2018.03.025

29. Harris, B. (2003). *When Your Kids Push Your Buttons and What You Can Do About It* (p. xxiii). New York: Warner Books.

30. MacKenzie, M. J., Nicklas, E., Waldfogel, J., & Brooks-Gunn, J. (2012). Corporal punishment and child behavioural and cognitive outcomes through 5 years of age: Evidence from a Contemporary Urban Birth Cohort Study, *Infant and Child Development, 21,* 3–33.

31. Gordon, L. (1988). *Heroes of Their Own Lives: The Politics and History of Family Violence* (p. 172). New York: Viking Penguin.

32. Holden, G. W., Coleman, S. M., & Schmidt, K. L. (1995). Why 3-year-old children get spanked: Parent and child determinants as reported by college-educated mothers. *Merrill-Palmer Quarterly, 41*(4), 431–452.

33. Lerner, H. (1998). *The Mother Dance*. New York: Harper Perennial.

34. Lerner, H. (1998). *The Mother Dance*. New York: Harper Perennial.

35. Gesell, A., & Ilg, F. A. (1946). *The Child From Five to Ten* (p. 411). New York: Harper & Row.

36. Konstantareas, M. M., & Desbois, N. (2001). Preschoolers' perceptions of the unfairness of maternal disciplinary practices. *Child Abuse & Neglect, 25,* 473–488.

37. Coontz, S. (1997). *The Way We Really Are: Coming to Terms With America's Changing Families*. New York: Basic Books.

38. Lerner, H. (1998). *The Mother Dance* (p. 126). New York: Harper Perennial.

39. Baum, W. M., & Kupfer, A. S. (2005). Behavior analysis, evolutionary theory, and the corporal discipline of children. In M. Donnelly & M. A. Straus (Eds.), *Corporal Punishment of Children in Theoretical Perspective* (pp. 103–133). New Haven, CT: Yale University Press.

40. Baum, W. M., & Kupfer, A. S. (2005). Behavior analysis, evolutionary theory, and the corporal discipline of children. In M. Donnelly & M. A. Straus (Eds.), *Corporal Punishment of Children in Theoretical Perspective* (pp. 103–133). New Haven, CT: Yale University Press.

41. Baum, W. M., & Kupfer, A. S. (2005). Behavior analysis, evolutionary theory, and the corporal discipline of children. In M. Donnelly & M. A. Straus (Eds.), *Corporal Punishment of Children in Theoretical Perspective* (pp. 103–133). New Haven, CT: Yale University Press.

42. Coontz, S. (1988). *The Social Origins of Private Life* (p. 2). New York: Verso.

43. Coates, T. (2015). *Between the World and Me*. New York: Spiegel & Grau.

44. Coates, T. (2015). *Between the World and Me* (p. 82). New York: Spiegel & Grau.

45. Menakem, R. (2017). *My Grandmother's Hands: Racialized Trauma and the Pathways to Mending Our Hearts and Bodies*. Las Vegas: Central Recovery Press.

46. Samalin, N. (1991). *Love and Anger: The Parental Dilemma* (p. 16). New York: Penguin.

47. Collins, R. (2005). Conflict theory of corporal punishment. In M. Donnelly & M. A. Straus (Eds.), *Corporal Punishment of Children in Theoretical Perspective* (p. 207). New Haven, CT: Yale University Press.

48. Shelov, S. P. (2009). *Caring for Your Young Baby and Child: Birth to Age 5* (p. 279). New York: Bantam Books.
49. Lerner, H. (1998). *The Mother Dance* (p. 224). New York: Harper Perennial.
50. Ansari, A., & Crosnoe, R. (2015). Children's elicitation of changes in parenting during the early childhood years. *Early Childhood Research Quarterly, 32,* 139–149.
51. Gesell, A., & Ilg, F.A. (1946). *The Child From Five to Ten* (p. 411). New York: Harper & Row.

Chapter 8

1. No Author. (1908). The spank annoyance. *Journal of Education, 68*(14), 402.
2. Brown, B. W. (1979). Parents' discipline of children in public places. *Family Coordinator, 28*(1), 67.
3. Rupkalvis, D. (2011, April 29). My-turn-as-for-me-I-will-spank-my-children. *The Graham Leader.* ACC-NO: 20110429-UI.
4. Carson, B. A. (1986). *Parents Who Don't Spank: Deviation in the Legitimation of Physical Force.* Doctoral Dissertation, University of New Hampshire.
5. Radl, S. L. (1980). American baby: To spank or not to Spank. *American Association for Maternal and Child Health, 42,* 42.
6. Gelles, R. J. (2005). Exchange theory. In M. Donnelly & M. A. Straus (Eds.), *Corporal Punishment of Children in Theoretical Perspective* (pp. 245–254). New Haven, CT: Yale University Press.
7. Ross, K., & Brock, S. (2018). Man arrested for spanking stranger's child in grocery store. https://www.wfmynews2.com/article/news/crime/man-arrested-for-spanking-strangers-child-in-grocery-store-checkout-line/83-516339847
8. Holden, G. W., Coleman, S. M., & Schmidt, K. L. (1995). Why 3-year-old children get spanked: Parent and child determinants as reported by college-educated mothers. *Merrill-Palmer Quarterly, 41*(4), 431–452.
9. Harris, B. (2003) *When Your Kids Push Your Buttons and What You Can Do About It* (p. 241).New York: Warner Books.
10. Kirkland, A. (2009). *Beating Black Kids: So What Have You Been Beat With?* New York: Asadah Sense Consulting. In her self-published book, Asadah bravely addresses many of the reasons parents hit their kids and shows the flaws in these beliefs.
11. Konstantareas, M. M., & Desbois, N. (2001). Pre-schoolers perceptions of the unfairness of maternal disciplinary practices. *Child Abuse & Neglect, 25,* 473–488.
12. Sheffield Morris, A., Silk, J. S., Steinberg, L., Sessa, F. M., Avenevoli, S., & Essex, M. J. (2002). Temperamental vulnerability and negative parenting as interacting predictors of child adjustment. *Journal of Marriage and Family, 64*(2), 461–471.
13. Guarendi, R.N. (1985). *You're a Better Parent Than You Think* (p. 2). Prentice Hall New York.
14. Brown, B. (2012). *Daring Greatly: How the Courage to Be Vulnerable Transforms the Way We Live, Love, Parent and Lead* (p. 215). New York: Gotham.
15. Dowrick, S. (2005). *Choosing Happiness: Life and Soul Essentials.* New York: Penguin.
16. This American Life. (August 11, 2019). National Public Radio: New York Public Radio.
17. *The Daily Show.* (2021, November 20). Trevor Noah interviews Dwyane Wade about embracing and championing a trans child.
18. Gershoff, E. T. (2016). Medical center staff attitudes about spanking. *Child Abuse& Neglect, 61,* 55–62.

19. Taylor, C. A., Fleckman, J. A., Scholer, S. J., & Branco, N. (2018). US pediatricians' attitudes, beliefs, and perceived injunctive norms about spanking. *Journal of Developmental & Behavioral Pediatrics, 39*(7), 564–572.

20. Burkhart, K., Knox, M., & Hunter, K. (2016). Changing healthcare professionals' attitudes towards spanking. *Clinical Pediatrics, 55*(11), 1005–1011.

21. The Quick Parenting Assessment can be accessed at https://www.childrenshospitalvanderb ilt.org/information/quick-parenting-assessment. The Play Nicely program can be found at https://www.childrenshospitalvanderbilt.org/information/play-nicely-healthy-discipline-program.

22. Hudnut-Beumler, J., Smith, A., & Scholer, S. J. (2018). How to convince parents to stop spanking their children. *Clinical Pediatrics, 57*(2), 129–136; Chavis. A., Hudnut-Beumler, J., Webb, M. W., Neely, J. A., Bickmand, L., Dietriche, M. S., & Scholer, S. J. (2013). A brief intervention affects parents' attitudes toward using less physical punishment. *Child Abuse & Neglect, 31*, 1192–1201. Burkhart, K., Knox, M., Hunter, K., Pennewitt, D., & Schrouder, K. (2018). Decreasing caregivers positive attitudes towards spanking. *Journal of Pediatric Health Care, 32*(4), 333–339.

23. Zolotor, A. (2014). Corporal punishment. *Pediatric Clinics of North America, 61*, 971–978.http://dx.doi.org/10.1016/j.pcl.2014.06.003

24. Taylor, C. A., Hamvas, L., Rice, J. C., Newman, D., & DeJong, W. (2011). Perceived social norms, expectations, and attitudes toward corporal punishment among an urban community sample of parents. *Journal of Urban Health, 88*(2), 254–269. http://dx.doi.org/10.1007/s11524-011-9548-7; and Taylor, C. A., Lee, S. J., Guterman, N. B., & Rice, J. C. (2010). Use of spanking for 3-year-old children and associated intimate partner aggression or violence. *Pediatrics, 126*(3), 415–424. https://doi.org/10.1542/peds.2010-0314

25. Healthy Children is the educational arm of the American Academy of Pediatrics. https://www.healthychildren.org/English/family-life/family-dynamics/communication-discipl ine/Pages/Where-We-Stand-Spanking.aspx

26. Davis, P. W. (1991, May). Stranger intervention into child punishment in public places. *Social Problems, 38*(2), 227–246.

27. Davis, P. W. (1991, May). stranger intervention into child punishment in public places. *Social Problems, 38*(2), 227–246

28. Katie, B. (2007). A thousand names for joy: Living in harmony with the way things are (pp. 76–77). New York: Harmony Books.

29. Casey, C. (2017). When child discipline crosses the line. *SoJust, 2*(1), 10–11, Saint Louis University College for Public Health and Social Justice.

30. Erickson, C. L., Gault, D., & Simmons, D. (2014). The Wakanheza Project: A public health approach to the primary prevention of family violence. *Journal of Community Practice, 22*, 1–15.

31. Pais, M. S. (2021). Placing children's freedom from violence at the heart of the policy agenda. In J. Todres & S. M. King (Eds.), *The Oxford Handbook of Children's Rights Law* (p. 307). New York: Oxford University Press.

32. Gagné, M. H., Tourigny, M., Joly, J., & Pouliot-Lapointe, J. (2007, October). Predictors of adult attitudes toward corporal punishment of children. *Journal of Interpersonal Violence, 22*(10), 1285–1304.

33. Maa, J., Grogan-Kaylorb, A., & Lee, S. J. (2018). Associations of neighborhood disorganization and maternal spanking with children's aggression: A fixed-effects regression analysis. *Child Abuse & Neglect, 76*, 106–116. https://doi.org/10.1016/j.chiabu.2017.10.013

34. *Love Them First: Lessons from Lucy Laney Elementary.* (2019). Award winning documentary film. https://www.lovethemfirst.com/

35. Bronfenbrenner, U. (2005). *Making Human Beings Human: Bioecological Perspectives on Human Development.* Thousand Oaks, CA: Sage; and Kemp, S. P., Whittaker, J. A., & Tracy, E. (1997). *Person-Environment Practice: The Social Ecology of Interpersonal Helping.* New York: Aldine de Gruyter.

36. Collins, R. (2005). Conflict theory of corporal punishment. In M. Donnelly & M. A. Straus (Eds.), *Corporal Punishment of Children in Theoretical Perspective* (pp. 199–213). New Haven, CT: Yale University Press.

37. Wilkins, N., Myers, L., Kuehl, T., Bauman, A., & Hertz, M. (2018). Connecting the Dots: State Health Department Approaches to Addressing Shared Risk and Protective Factors Across Multiple Forms of Violence. *Journal of Public Health Management Practice, 24*(Suppl.), 32–41.

Chapter 9

1. Brown, B. (2012). *Daring Greatly: How the Courage to be Vulnerable Transforms the Way We Live, Love, Parent, and Lead* (p. 214). New York: Gotham.

2. Miller, D. R., & Swanson G. E. (1958). *The Changing American Parent* (p. 236). New York: John Wiley and Sons

3. Giles-Sims, J., & Lockhart, C. (2005). Grid group theory and corporal punishment. In M. Donnelly & M. A. Straus (Eds.), *Corporal Punishment of Children in Theoretical Perspective* (pp. 55–71). New Haven: Yale University Press.

4. *Minneapolis Star-Tribune.* (2018, November 11). Readers write, spanking, look, it worked for us.

5. Leman, K., & Carlson, R. (1993). *Parent Talk: Straight Answers to the Questions That Rattle Moms and Dads* (p. 35). Nashville, TN: Nelson.

6. Mogel, W. (2010). *The Blessings of a B Minus: Using Jewish Teachings to Raise Resilient Teenagers* (pp. 73–75). New York: Scribner.

7. Ekman, P. (2010, June 21). Paul Ekman's taxonomy of compassion. The Greater Good Science Center at the University of California, Berkeley. https://greatergood.berkeley.edu/article/item/paul_ekmans_taxonomy_of_compassion

8. Schilder, P. (1950). *Image and Appearance of the Human Body.* New York: International Universities Press.

9. Stack, D. M., & Muir, D. W. (1992). Adult tactile stimulation during face-to-face interactions modulates five-month-olds' affect and attention. *Child Development, 63,* 1509–1525.

10. Blaesing, S., & Brockhaus, J. (1972). The development of body image in the child. *Nursing Clinician in North America. 7*(4), 597–607.

11. Barnard, K. E., & Brazelton, T. B. (1990) *Touch: The Foundation of Experience* (p. 196). Madison, CT: International Universities Press.

12. Aznar, A., & Tenenbaum, H. R. (2016). Parent-child positive touch: Gender, age and task differences. *Journal of Nonverbal Behavior, 40,* 317–333.

13. Gerhardt, S. (2004). *Why Love Matters: How Affection Shapes a Babies Brain.* New York: Brunner-Routledge.

14. Stansbury, K., Haley, D., Lee, J., & Brophy-Herb, H. E. (2012). Adult caregivers behavioural responses to child noncompliance in public settings: Gender differences and the role of positive and negative touch. *Behavior and Social Issues, 21*, 80–114.

15. Infante, D. A. (2005). Corporal punishment of children: A communication theory perspective. In M. Donnelly & M. A. Straus (Eds.), *Corporal Punishment of Children in Theoretical Perspective* (pp. 183–198). New Haven: Yale University Press.

16. Infante, D. A. (2005). Corporal punishment of children: A communication theory perspective. In M. Donnelly & M. A. Straus (Eds.), *Corporal Punishment of Children in Theoretical Perspective* (pp. 183–198). New Haven: Yale University Press.

17. Infante, D. A. (2005). Corporal punishment of children: A communication theory perspective. In M. Donnelly & M. A. Straus (Eds.), *Corporal Punishment of Children in Theoretical Perspective* (pp. 183–198). New Haven: Yale University Press.

18. Collins, R. (2005). Conflict theory of corporal punishment. In M. Donnelly & M. A. Straus (Eds.), *Corporal Punishment of Children in Theoretical Perspective* (pp. 199–213). New Haven: Yale University Press.

19. Van Der Kolk, B. (2014). *The Body Keeps the Score. Brain, Mind and Body in the Healing of Trauma*. New York: Viking.

20. Greven, P. J. (1990). *Spare the Child: The Religious Roots of Punishment and the Psychological Impact of Physical Abuse* (p. 7). New York: Vintage Books.

21. Menakem, R. (2017). *My Grandmother's Hands: Racialized Trauma and the Pathways to Mending Our Hearts and Bodies* (p. 7). Las Vegas: Central Recovery Press.

22. Menakem, R. (2017). *My Grandmother's Hands: Racialized Trauma and the Pathway to Mending Our Hearts and Bodies*. Las Vegas: Central Recovery Press.

23. Menakem, R. (2017). *My Grandmother's Hands: Racialized Trauma and the Pathway to Mending Our Hearts and Bodies*. Las Vegas: Central Recovery Press.

24. Hemenway, D., Solnick, S., & Carter, J. (1994). Child rearing violence. *Child Abuse & Neglect, 18*(12), 1011–1020.

25. Hite, S. (1994). *The Hite Report on the Family: Growing Up Under Patriarchy*. New York: Grove Press.

26. Hugh Missildine, W. (1963). *Your Inner Child of the Past*. New York: Simon & Schuster.

27. Leman, K. (2007). *What Your Childhood Memories Say About You and What You Can Do About It*. Carol Stream, IL: Tyndale House Publishers.

28. Van Der Kolk, B. (2014). *The Body Keeps the Score. Brain, Mind and Body in the Healing of Trauma* (p. 129). New York: Viking.

29. Menakem, R. (2017). *My Grandmother's Hands: Racialized Trauma and the Pathway to Mending Our Hearts and Bodies*. Las Vegas: Central Recovery Press.

30. Goleman, D. (2006). *Social Intelligence: The New Science of Human Relationships* (p. 152). New York: Bantam.

31. Gerhardt, S. (2004) *Why Love Matters: How Affection Shapes a Baby's Brain*. New York: Brunner-Routledge.

32. Anderson, J. (2021, April 13). The effect of spanking on the brain. Harvard Graduate School of Education. Usable Knowledge. https://www.gse.harvard.edu/news/uk/21/04/effect-spanking-brain

33. Cuartas, J., McCoy, D. C., Grogan-Kaylor, A., & Gershoff, E. (2020). Physical punishment as a predictor of early cognitive development: Evidence from econometric approaches. *Developmental Psychology, 56*(11), 2013–2026.

34. Tomoda, A., Yi-Shin Sheu, B. S., Keren Rabi, M. A., Hanako Suzuki, M. A., Navalta, C. P., Polcari, A., & Teicher, M. H. (2009). Reduced prefrontal cortical gray matter volume in young adults exposed to harsh corporal punishment. *NeuroImage, 47*, T66–T71.

35. Cuartas, J., Weissman, D. G., Sheridan, M. A., Lengua, L., & McLaughlin, K. A. (2021). Corporal punishment and elevated neural response to threat in children. *Child Development, 92*(3), 821–832. https://doi.org/10.1111/cdev.13565

36. Pace, G. T., Lee, S. J., & Grogan-Kaylor, A. (2019). Spanking and young children's socioemotional development in low- and middle-income countries. *Child Abuse & Neglect, 88*, 84–95. https://doi.org/10.1016/j.chiabu.2018.11.003

37. Bennet, R. P. (2013, November 23). Violence: A family tradition. *Ted Talk.* https://www.yout ube.com/watch?v=WLMJHdySgE8&list=PLg8k0xDP36cx7BZRp0u_wElGUiRNibTtt

38. Davis, M., et. al. (2018). A systematic review of parent–child synchrony: It is more than skin deep. Developmental psychobiology. *International Society for Developmental Psychobiology, 60*(6), 674–691.

39. Tronick, E. Z. (1989). Emotions and emotional communication in infants. *American Psychologist, 44*(2), 112.

40. Goleman, D. (2006). *Social Intelligence: The New Science of Human Relationships.* New York: Bantam.

41. Van Der Kolk, B. (2014). *The Body Keeps the Score. Brain, Mind and Body in the Healing of Trauma.* New York: Viking.

42. Goleman, D. (2006). *Social Intelligence: The New Science of Human Relationships.* Bantam: New York.

43. Goleman, D. (2006). *Social Intelligence: The New Science of Human Relationships.* Bantam: New York.

44. Van Der Kolk, B. (2014). *The Body Keeps the Score. Brain, Mind and Body in the Healing of Trauma.* New York: Viking.

45. Bugental, D. B., Martorell, G. A., & Barraza, V. (2003). The hormonal costs of subtle forms of infant maltreatment. *Hormones and Behavior, 43*(1), 237–244.

46. Center for the Developing Child, Harvard University. https://developingchild.harvard.edu/resources/what-is-epigenetics-and-how-does-it-relate-to-child-development/

47. *TedMed.* (2014). How childhood trauma affects health across a lifetime. https://www.ted.com/talks/nadine_burke_harris_how_childhood_trauma_affects_health_across_a_lifetime?referrer=playlist-how_does_my_brain_work&language=en#t-328343

48. Ackerman, D.(1985). *A Natural History of Love* (p. 151). New York: Random House.

49. Felitti, V. J., Anda, R. F., Nordenberg, D., Williamson, D. F., Spitz, A. M., Edwards, V., Koss, M. P., & Marks, J. S. (1998). Relationship of childhood abuse and household dysfunction to many of the leading causes of death in adults: The Adverse Childhood Experiences (ACE) Study. *American Journal of Preventive Medicine, 14*(4), 245–258.https://doi.org/10.1016/S0749-3797(98)00017-8

50. Afifi, T. O., Ford, D., Gershoff, E. T., Merrick, M., Grogan-Kaylor, A., Ports, K. A., MacMillan, H. L., Holden, G. W., Taylor, C. A., Lee, S. J., & Bennett, R. P. (2017). Spanking and adult mental health impairment: The case for the designation of spanking as an adverse childhood experience, *Child Abuse & Neglect, 71*, 24–31. https://doi.org/10.1016/j.chiabu.2017.01.014; Afifi, T. O. (2020). Considerations for expanding the definition of ACE's. In Asmundson, G. (Ed.), *Adverse Childhood Experiences: Using Evidence to Advance Research, Practice, Policy and Prevention.* London: Elsevier Academic Press.

51. Afifi, T. O., Ford, D., Gershoff, E. T., Merrick, M., Grogan-Kaylor, A., Ports, K. A., MacMillan, H. L., Holden, G. W., Taylor, C. A., Lee, S. J., & Bennett, R. P. (2017). Spanking and adult mental health impairment: The case for the designation of spanking as an adverse childhood experience, *Child Abuse & Neglect, 71*, 24–31. https://doi.org/10.1016/j.chiabu.2017.01.014

52. Thoits, P. A. (2010). Stress and health: Major findings and policy implications. *Journal of Health and Social Behavior, 51*(Suppl.), S41–S53.

53. Hite, S. (1994). *The Hite Report on the Family: Growing Up Under Patriarchy*. New York: Grove Press.

54. Lansford, J. E., Wager, L. B., Bates, J. E., Pettit, G. S., & Dodge, K. A. (2012, April). Forms of spanking and children's externalizing behaviors. *Family Relations, 61*(2), 224–236.

55. Infante, D. A. (2005). Corporal punishment of children: A communication theory perspective. In M. Donnelly & M. A. Straus (Eds.), *Corporal Punishment of Children in Theoretical Perspective* (pp. 183–198). New Haven: Yale University Press.

56. Garrett-Akinsanya, B. V. (2017). The Importance of parenting for highly stressed children and families. Presentation Sponsored by the University of Minnesota Institute for Translational Research Minneapolis, MN. https://www.youtube.com/watch?v=KFNepnvOZAQ.

57. Lerner, H. (1998). *The Mother Dance* (p. 121). New York: Harper Perennial.

58. Patton, S. (2017). *Spare the Kids: Why Whupping Children Won't Save Black America*. Boston: Beacon Press.

59. Holden, G. W., Coleman, S. M., & Schmidt, K. L. (1995). Why 3-year-old children get spanked: Parent and child determinants as reported by college-educated mothers. *Merrill-Palmer Quarterly, 41*(4), 431–452.

60. Menakem, R. (2017). *My Grandmother's Hands: Racialized Trauma and the Pathway to Mending Our Hearts and Bodies*. Las Vegas: Central Recovery Press.

61. Infante, D. A. (2005). Corporal punishment of children: A communication theory perspective. In M. Donnelly & M. A. Straus (Eds.), *Corporal Punishment of Children in Theoretical Perspective* (pp. 183–198). New Haven: Yale University Press.

62. Infante, D. A. (2005). Corporal punishment of children: A communication theory perspective. In M. Donnelly & M. A. Straus (Eds.), *Corporal Punishment of Children in Theoretical Perspective* (pp. 183–198). New Haven: Yale University Press.

63. Samalin, N. (1991). *Love and Anger: The Parental Dilemma* (p. 4). New York: Penguin Books.

64. Coontz, S. (1992). *The Way We Never Were: American Families and the Nostalgia Trap*. New York: Basic Books.

65. Coontz, S. (1992). *The Way We Never Were: American Families and the Nostalgia Trap*. New York: Basic Books.

66. Furnham, A. (2005). Spare the rod and spoil the child: lay theories of corporal punishment. In M. Donnelly & M. A. Straus (Eds.), *Corporal Punishment of Children in Theoretical Perspective* (pp. 134–150). New Haven: Yale University Press.

67. Brown, B. (2012). *Daring Greatly: How the Courage to be Vulnerable Transforms the Way We Live, Love, Parent, and Lead* (pp. 229–230). New York: Gotham.

68. Mogel, W. (2010). *Blessings of a B Minus: Using Jewish Teachings to Raise Resilient Teenagers* (p. 225). New York: Scribner.

69. Guarendi, R. N. (1985). *You're a Better Parent Than You Think! A Guide to Common Sense Parenting* (p. 30). New York: Prentice Hall.

70. Korbin, J. E., & Krugman, R. D. (2015). *Child Maltreatment: Contemporary Issues in Research and Policy.* New York: Springer.

Chapter 10

1. Chapin, H. (1972). Lyrics from *Cats in the Cradle.* http://www.songlyrics.com/harry-chapin/cat-s-in-the-cradle-lyrics/

2. Moyers, B. (1988). E. L. Doctorow on the role of writers in society. https://billmoyers.com/content/e-l-doctorow-best-writers/

3. Taja, F., & Baker-Henningham, H. (2020). Design and implementation of the Irie Homes Toolbox: A violence prevention, early childhood, parenting program. *Frontiers in Public Health, 8,* 702. https://www.frontiersin.org/article/10.3389/fpubh.2020.582961 and www.zerotothree.org

4. Day, D. E., & Roberts M. W. (1983). An analysis of the physical punishment component of a parent training program. *Journal of Abnormal Child Psychology, 11*(1), 141–152; Warzak, W. J., & Floress, M. T. (2009). Time-out training without put-backs, spanks or restraint: A brief report of deferred time out. *Child and Family Behavior Therapy, 31,* 134–143; Everett, G. E., Hupp, S. D. A., & Olmi, D. J. (2010). Time-out with parents: A descriptive analysis of 30 years of research. *Education and Treatment of Children, 33*(2), 235–259.

5. Meghji, R. (2021). *Every Conversation Counts.* Vancouver, BC: Page Two Books.

6. Pais, M. S. (2021). Placing children's freedom from violence at the heart of the policy agenda. In J. Todres & S. M. King (Eds.), *The Oxford Handbook of Children's Rights Law* (p. 307). New York: Oxford University Press.

7. Coontz, S. (1992) *The Way We Never Were: American Families and the Nostalgia Trap.* New York: Basic Books.

8. Goodman, L. (2021, November). The best defense: Paul K. Chappell on the urgent need for peace literacy. *The Sun.* https://thesunmagazine.org/

9. Corporal punishment of children and public health: What does the research tell us? (.2021, October 5). Webinar hosted jointly by End Violence Against Children and the World Health Organization. https://endcorporalpunishment.org/corporal-punishment-and-public-health-what-does-research-tell-us/

10. Straus, M., & Donnelly, D. A. (2009). *Beating the Devil Out of Them: Corporal Punishment in American Families and Its Effects on Children.* New Brunswick, NJ: Transaction Publishers.

11. Hering, K. (2021, January). Authority. *Community, 44*(5), 1. Unity Church Unitarian.)

Book Group Questions

1. Bellah, R. N., Madsen, R., Sullivan, W. M., Swidler, A., & Tipton, S. M. (1985). *Habits of the Heart: Individualism and Commitment in Everyday Life* (pp. 132–133). New York: Harper & Row..

Index

For the benefit of digital users, indexed terms that span two pages (e.g., 52–53) may, on occasion, appear on only one of those pages.

Tables are indicated by *t* following the page number